Mature Beyond Their Years: The Impact of Cancer on Adolescent Development

Kathleen L. Neville, PhD, RN

with a contribution by Mary McElwain Petriccione, RN, MSN, PNP

D1509729

Oncology Nursing Press, Inc.
A subsidiary of the Oncology Nursing Society
Pittsburgh, PA

Oncology Nursing Press, Inc.
Publisher: Leonard Mafrica, MBA, CAE
Director of Commercial Publications: Barbara Sigler, RN, MNEd
Technical Editor: Dorothy Mayernik, RN, MSN
Staff Editor: Lisa M. George, BA
Copy Editor: Jason Snyder, BA
Creative Services Assistant: Dany Sjoen

Funding for this book was partially supported by a grant from Kean University Office of Grants.

Mature Beyond Their Years: The Impact of Cancer on Adolescent Development

Copyright © 2000 by the Oncology Nursing Press, Inc.

All rights reserved. No part of the material protected by this copyright may be reproduced or utilized in any form, electronic or mechanical, including photocopying, recording, or by an information storage and retrieval system, without written permission from the copyright owner. For information, write to the Oncology Nursing Press, Inc., 501 Holiday Drive, Pittsburgh, PA 15220-2749.

Library of Congress Card Catalog Number: 00-107539

ISBN 1-890504-20-3

Publisher's Note
This book is published by the Oncology Nursing Press, Inc. (ONP). ONP neither represents nor guarantees that the practices described herein will, if followed, ensure safe and effective patient care. The recommendations contained in this manual reflect ONP's judgment regarding the state of general knowledge and practice in the field as of the date of publication. The recommendations may not be appropriate for use in all circumstances. Those who use this book should make their own determinations regarding specific safe and appropriate patient-care practices, taking into account the personnel, equipment, and practices available at the hospital or other facility at which they are located. The editors and publisher cannot be held responsible for any liability incurred as a consequence from the use or application of any of the contents of these guidelines. Figures and tables are used as examples only. They are not meant to be all-inclusive, nor do they represent endorsement of any particular institution by the Oncology Nursing Society (ONS). Mention of specific products and opinions related to those products do not indicate or imply endorsement by ONS or ONP.

ONS and ONP publications are originally published in English. Permission has been granted by the ONS Board of Directors for foreign translation. (Individual tables and figures that are reprinted or adapted require additional permission from the original source.) However, because translations from English may not always be accurate and precise, ONS and ONP disclaim any responsibility for inaccurate translations. Readers relying on precise information should check the original English version.

Printed in the United States of America

Oncology Nursing Press, Inc.
A subsidiary of the Oncology Nursing Society

To the men in my life—
Cap, Jackie, Michael, and Thomas

Table of Contents

Foreword

Adolescents, Human Development, and Cancer

As clinicians and scientists, nurses have interpreted the behavior and problem solving of adolescents within the context of several widely accepted theories of human development. Kathleen L. Neville, PhD, RN, succinctly summarizes these theories, which lead into her descriptions of the impact of cancer on adolescent development. Neville positions her readers to question the usefulness of these theories in relating to adolescents who are experiencing a potentially life-threatening illness—cancer—and its life-changing treatments. These theories, which are based entirely on the observations of well children, propose that human development is linear and occurring in sequential stages. Do linear-stage theories adequately depict the social, mental, emotional, and spiritual development of adolescents who experience cancer? The test of the appropriateness of the theories lies in clinical care: Do these theories give accurate guidance to nurses and other healthcare professionals who seek to give age- and event-sensitive care to adolescents with cancer? Or are the theories limited in their application to adolescents who are ill, serving primarily to identify how these adolescents differ from their healthy peers? As adolescents realize that cancer threatens their existence, how does that realization alter their social, mental, emotional, and spiritual dimensions and the expression of those dimensions? Does their response to cancer create new dimensions? Do adolescents with cancer then experience more or less stages of development and spend more or less time within a given stage than their well peers, or is the process of development nonlinear for adolescents during their experience with cancer and then linear after the cancer experience? If development is altered, is the alteration durable?

Existing theories of human development do not consistently reflect gender or biological differences (Asendorpf & Valsiner, 1992; Belenky, Clinchy, Goldberger, & Tarule, 1986; Brodie, 1998; Gilligan, 1982; Kindlon & Thompson, 1999) or health differences (Blumberg, Lewis, & Susman, 1984; Muuss, 1996). Both Neville and Mary McElwain-Petriccione, RN, MSN, PNP, offer powerful descriptions of the intense treatment that adolescents with cancer must tolerate in an effort to achieve cure. The treatment alters adolescents' biological and genetic makeup and their physiological and psychosocial processes. That such intense treatments have no impact on an evolving process such as human development, which is known to be sensitive to external influences, is difficult to imagine. Is the impact such that it interrupts development, speeds development, or changes its form altogether? If we perceive and interpret the impact of cancer on adolescent development through theories that do not truly reflect the cancer experience, we will never know their real impact.

If we, as clinicians, apply theories or, as scientists, interpret data in light of certain theories, but the theories do not adequately represent our target group, we will not be able to provide age-specific care and risk misinterpreting data. To minimize such risks, we must question what has been so widely accepted and do so with clinical and scientific data. Nurses are equipped with the clinical skills to observe for alterations in human development, have the opportunity to make such observations, and have the caring curiosity to pursue the question of the impact of cancer on adolescent development. Nurses and their colleagues are actively seeking experience- and data-based guidance on the best ways to give care to adolescents—the kind of care that supports their development in the midst of a most unusual life situation. Neville emphasizes the importance of listening to adolescents with cancer to learn what their cancer means to them and to use what we hear to provide the basis for highest quality nursing care. This action alone is worthwhile, but we also could, through both listening to what patients say and through observation, determine if current theories of human development represent adolescents with cancer or if new theoretical perspectives are needed to better guide health care for adolescents. A different theoretical perspective could have huge implications for how we define age-appropriate health care for adolescents. We may have to change the ways in which we relate to adolescents. Should we direct our care toward prolonging or abbreviating certain developmental aspects of the adolescents' responses to cancer and its treatment—do we attempt to speed or slow their responses in order to facilitate their development? Let us use our clinical and research skills and find out.

Asendorpf, J., & Valsiner, J. (1992). Three dimensions of developmental perspectives. In J.B. Asendorpf & J. Valsiner (Eds.), *Stability and change in development: A study of methodological reasoning* (pp. ix–xxii). Newbury Park, CA: Sage.

Belenky, M.F., Clinchy, B.M., Goldberger, N.R., & Tarule, J.M. (1986). *Women's ways of knowing: The development of self, voice, and mind.* New York: Basic Books, Inc.

Blumberg, B.D., Lewis, M.J., & Susman, E.J. (1984). Adolescence: A time of transition. In M.G. Eisenberg, L.C. Sutkin, & M.A. Jansen (Eds.), *Chronic illness and disability through the life span: Effects on self and family* (pp. 133–149). New York: Springer.

Brodie, B. (1998). Historical overview of health promotion for children and families in late 19th- and 20th-century America. In M. Broome, K. Knafl, K. Pridham, & S. Feetham (Eds.), *Children and families in health and illness* (pp. 3–14). Thousand Oaks, CA: Sage.

Gilligan, C. (1982). *In a different voice: Psychological theory and women's development.* Cambridge, MA: Harvard University Press.

Kindlon, D., & Thompson, M. (1999). *Raising Cain: Protecting the emotional lives of boys.* New York: Ballantine Books.

Muuss, R.E. (1996). *Theories of adolescence* (6th ed.). New York: McGraw-Hill.

Pamela S. Hinds, PhD, RN, CS
Director of Patient Care Services
St. Jude Children's Research Hospital
Memphis, TN

Preface

At some level, I like to think of this text as a celebration of nursing and even as a celebration of my own nursing career as a pediatric nurse engaged in practice, education, and research. I chose to write this text because of the rich experiences gained in nursing, and I believe the cumulative experience of the three interwoven domains of nursing inspired me to formulate this text. As nurses, we are so privileged to experience the diverse phenomena we see in practice as we work with individuals and families of all backgrounds and histories. Similar to the findings that will be discussed in this book regarding survivors of teenage cancer, nurses, I believe, also possess a mature way of thinking that, in many cases, is far beyond their chronologic years. As a result of all the difficult realities and hardships that nurses witness while providing care to all types of patients and families in all types of settings, many nurses develop mature values, explore existential meaning in life, and have a strong appreciation for the fragility of life.

I know for certain that my clinical experiences have formidably shaped my life. The host of clinical experiences that I have witnessed and participated in throughout the years have influenced the manner in which I determine what is important to me, the way in which I raise my children, and even my worries and concerns. Our experiences in clinical practice are by no means commonplace. They can be extremely demanding and exhausting yet tremendously exciting, fulfilling, and challenging. Our experiences and stories should be documented or shared more frequently, and the full range of our comprehensive roles should be communicated more descriptively so that a more accurate picture of the art and science of scholarly nursing is more globally recognized. This book, in essence, is a tribute to nurses for what they do and, perhaps, do not articulate.

Nurses face challenging demands every day of their practice, and few would argue about the demands and rigor involved in working with children with cancer. One of the recurring thoughts that I have had as I wrote this book has to do with the developmental processes of nurses and the impact of their chronologic age on their own practices. Although the mean age for practicing nurses has increased to approximately 40, many nurses enter practice in their second decade of life as young adults or even as late adolescents. I remember that when I began to practice in pediatric cancer nursing, many of the nurses were similar in age to the patients who were in late adolescence or young adulthood. I would now venture to say that few nurses, as they progress in age, remain in inpatient oncology units as staff nurses, but I question how their practice would differ as they aged. Working with children and adolescents with potentially life-threatening illness requires great strength, perseverance, and resilience as well as maturity. As I conducted postdoctoral research on clinical units and interacted with adolescents, I often reflected on how my advanced age (as compared to 20 years ago) and increased maturity gained throughout the years would affect my interventions with ill adolescents if I remained exclusively in clinical practice today. Would I be more receptive to discussing volatile issues? Would I have a better understanding of death and dying of children and adolescents? I have no answers to these questions, but I would like to acknowledge the fortitude and strength of young oncology nurses who so readily accept and deal with these tremendous responsibilities at such an early time in their lives. I also know that it was one of the most exciting times in my career and a time that I cherished. While conducting research and resuming contact with adolescents and families, I realized how much I missed this contact and how much of the pleasure and fulfillment of nursing comes from working directly with adolescents and their families.

During the formulation of this book, I reflected on the collective group of nurse colleagues that I worked with as a beginning pediatric nurse and who helped me to develop skill and expertise in my professional nursing practice. Pediatric oncology practice was not as optimistic in 1978 as it is now because mortality rates among adolescents with cancer were dramatically higher. This special cohort of nurses, individually and collectively, functioned superbly in the face of crises and losses and influenced my career path in nursing. Those rich experiences and later experiences influenced my desire to share my expertise in the psychosocial responses of adolescents with cancer.

My strong interest in formulating this text has evolved from my clinical experiences and research devoted to adolescents with cancer. My principal research interest lies in the area of psychosocial responses to cancer during adolescence. I now have completed research on the psychosocial responses to illness during the diagnostic phase of cancer and, most recently, when surviving cancer five or more years after diagnosis. Although my research findings will serve as a source for my writing, the text will not be a research document. Instead, it will focus on the unique experience of living through and surviving cancer and addressing the issues and concerns faced by adolescents surviving a malignancy. Special emphasis will be placed on how cancer impacts the developmental tasks of adolescence.

The book is actually an evolutionary process and was not developed entirely by me. The idea for this book solidified when I was conducting an interview with a young adult who had survived leukemia during her early teen years. This intense interview focused on how cancer affected her development, and she described many common survivorship issues and concerns, such as social isolation, reduced stamina, poor health, and feelings of being different from others. After identifying these findings repeatedly in previous interviews with other survivors, I revealed to her that her responses were not unusual but, in fact, quite typical reactions to surviving cancer. Her favorable response was dramatic and immediate and revealed incredible relief. In addition, she, like all other survivors interviewed, identified how appreciative she was to have the opportunity to "talk through" her cancer experience years later and how having the continued opportunity to freely and openly discuss her cancer experience is necessary. Part of this openness of communication may be related to young adults' willingness to participate in this research so that other survivors can benefit from the research findings. The fact that I had not been involved in the care of for these adolescents and survivors may have influenced the "free and open" communication patterns of the interviews. They perceived that they could speak their minds freely and without any concern for their families' or even staff responses regarding their comments.

That poignant interview with one memorable survivor was the real impetus for this work. As I left the interview, I recognized the strong need to communicate these common findings that, unfortunately at the time of the interview, she thought were so abnormal and pathological.

During these interviews, the participants revealed many common responses to cancer, but, most importantly, they exhibited tremendous relief when I shared with them how universal these responses were. Several common themes were identified. Survivors reported feeling dramatically different from others who did not have a cancer experience. All described the importance of catching up academically and socially. Peer and family relations were another important focus of the interviews, and they described a self-transcendence toward a new and higher order of life.

The communication of these findings is vital to the care of adolescents and young adults in oncology practice today. As increasing numbers of young people survive cancer, addressing the psychosocial issues and concerns of adolescents and young adults assumes greater importance. This book will provide scientific knowledge and documentation of the continued need for the psychosocial assessment of survivors of adolescent cancer, thus contributing to the scarcity of literature about recovery from adolescent cancer.

This text will be clinically relevant for nurses and other healthcare professionals who are engaged in cancer practice. Understanding what I believe are universal psychosocial sequelae of cancer and discussing these issues with survivors are vital to the provision of holistic, comprehensive care.

Chapter 1, "Developmental Issues of Adolescence," provides an overview of adolescence, with emphasis on the normal developmental tasks of adolescence. The work of classic theorists such as G. Stanley Hall, Harry Stack Sullivan, Erik Erikson, and Sigmund Freud will be used in describing the period of adolescence. Attention will focus on Erikson and the importance of the acquisition of developmental tasks for adolescents.

Chapter 2, "Psychosocial Issues of Seriously Ill Adolescents," focuses on literature that deals with the challenges that adolescents and their families face when illness is superimposed on normal adolescent development. The psychosocial aspects of illness, adolescents' responses to serious and potentially life-threatening illnesses, protective communication patterns with family members, information seeking, and social issues will be addressed.

Chapter 3, "Overview of Cancer in Children and Adolescents," was written by Mary McElwain-Petriccione, RN, MSN, PNP, a longtime nurse colleague and expert advanced practice pediatric oncology nurse practitioner. As anyone who has had the privilege to work with Mary McElwain-Petriccione will attest, she exemplifies excellence in nursing. She possesses the extraordinary gifts of kindness, good will, compassion, intelligence, and expert knowledge in caring for children and adolescents with cancer.

This chapter will provide a broad overview of the state of the art in pediatric oncology and focuses on current treatment modalities for the most common forms of childhood and adolescent malignancies.

Chapter 4, "The Survivorship Movement," begins by addressing today's increased number of people who are surviving and living longer with cancer. Using the classic works by Susan Leigh, RN, BSN, and Fitzhugh Mullan, MD, about the phases of survivorship, the concept of survivorship will be described. The National Coalition for Cancer Survivorship will be introduced in this chapter, and its mission and purpose will be described. Issues relating to surviving cancer (e.g., personal relations, employment, disability, school) will be addressed.

Chapter 5, "Surviving Cancer During Adolescence," deals with the unique aspects of surviving cancer during adolescence. The themes identified by survivors of adolescent cancer including catching up academically and socially, are highlighted descriptively. The sense of being different and transcending to a new, higher order of life is addressed. Actual stories reported to me during my research will portray peer and family relations. The strength and resilience of survivors will be noted in this chapter. Common themes of concern for others, mature thinking, spirituality and transcendence, and focused career development will be highlighted.

Chapter 6, "The Role of Helping Cancer Survivors," concludes the book by addressing the need for healthcare professionals to continue to provide psychosocial support to survivors of adolescent cancer. The research of Diane Scott-Dorsett, RN, PhD, FAAN, which examines the trajectory of cancer and offers a new recovery model, highlights the need for continued psychosocial assessment long after cancer treatment ends.

This book is intended to portray in the best way possible cancer's impact on adolescent development for this small group of survivors and to share the commonalities of these findings to ultimately affect how the challenging discipline of cancer nursing of children and adolescents is practiced.

Kathleen L. Neville, PhD, RN

Acknowledgments

In memory of Inez Cosentino and Marion Petriccione, both of whom were incredible survivors of cancer who were unique and special and are missed immensely by their families. Both survivors succumbed to their illness during the summer, when great attention was focused on completing this text. Throughout the writings and during many days, they were thought of and fondly remembered for their kindness and contributions to others.

Introduction

Advances in biomedical science and technology have dramatically altered the course of cancer for many children and adolescents who are faced with the potentially life-threatening disease. During a period of approximately 25 years, childhood and adolescent cancer has evolved from an inevitably fatal illness to a potentially life-threatening, chronic disease.

Within industrialized Western countries, pediatric and adolescent cancers represent only 2% of cancers (Robinson, 1997). Despite that percentage, cancer is still the leading cause of death from disease for children 1–15 years of age.

Types and distributions of pediatric cancers are different than adult malignancies. However, contributions from pediatric cancer research have provided a substantial understanding of cancer, particularly in the field of genetics.

Although cancer has been documented to have existed for centuries, only since the latter part of the 20th century have tremendous strides been made in pediatric and adult cancers. Prior to World War II, the predominant treatment modalities were surgery and radiation. Paul Ehrlich, at the turn of the century, began the search for the "magic bullet," termed "chemotherapy" (Yarbro, 1992). Seamen exposed to nitrogen mustard gas as part of chemical warfare during World War II paved the way for the use of chemotherapy in treating cancer. Exposure to this gas led to the observation that alkylating agents cause bone marrow and lymphoid hypoplasia, which led to their use in humans in subsequent years (DeVita, 1993).

In the late 1940s, children began undergoing chemotherapy for cancer (Foley & Fergusson, 1993). Major strides in progress did not occur until pediatric oncology experts collaborated and interdisciplinary approaches were used. Until that time, cancer was associated with death. For years, the cancer care environment was one of protective withholding of information in which children and even adults were not informed of their illness and the word "cancer" was never spoken.

In 1960, less than 5% of children survived acute lymphocytic leukemia (ALL), but by 1991, five-year survival rates for ALL approached 60% (Jackson & Saunders, 1993). Child mortality rates have declined by 57% since the early 1970s (American Cancer Society, 1999).

The scientific advances in pediatric cancer have dramatically improved survival outcomes for children and adolescents with cancer. As the life prognosis for adolescents with cancer improves, the unique survivorship concerns and issues for this population assume a more salient role for those involved in caring for them.

References

American Cancer Society. (1999). *Cancer facts and figures, 1999*. Atlanta: Author.

DeVita, V. T. (1993). Principles of chemotherapy. In V.T. DeVita, S. Hellman, & S.A. Rosenberg (Eds.), *Cancer: Principles and practice of oncology* (4th ed.) (pp. 276–292). Philadelphia: J.B. Lippincott.

Foley, G.V., & Fergusson, J.M. (1993). History, issues and trends. In G.V. Foley, D. Fochtman, & K.H. Mooney (Eds.), *Nursing care of the child with cancer* (2nd ed.) (pp. 1–24). Philadelphia: W.B. Saunders.

Jackson, C., & Saunders, R. (1993). Children with cancer. In C. Jackson & R. Saunders (Eds.), *Child health nursing: A comprehensive approach to the care of children and their families* (pp. 731–759). Philadelphia: J.B. Lippincott.

Robinson, L.L. (1997). General principles of the epidemiology of childhood cancer. In P.A. Pizzo & D.G. Poplack (Eds.), *Principles and practice of pediatric oncology* (3rd ed.) (pp. 1–10). Philadelphia: Lippincott Raven.

Yarbro, J. (1992). The scientific basis of cancer chemotherapy. In M.C. Perry (Ed.), *The chemotherapy source book* (pp. 2–10). Baltimore: Williams & Wilkins.

CHAPTER 1.
Developmental Issues of Adolescence

Kathleen L. Neville, PhD, RN

Introduction

Adolescence is a complex time in life. Few people would refute the difficulties that are associated with this tumultuous period. This growth stage brings much excitement, discovery, and achievement; however, parents can attest to the many challenges inherent to a family with teenagers. A multitude of physiologic, cognitive, emotional, and social processes are incorporated in the transcendence from childhood to young adulthood. The dynamics register on both positive and negative scales: life is marked by accelerated growth and development, but it also is characterized by substantial turmoil and stress. Both adolescents and their families experience this stress. Healthcare professionals who work with this distinctive family unit play an important role in assisting parents and adolescents to understand the complexities of this transitional period and optimally manage the unique stressors they will confront during these years.

The nurse's role as educator is important to healthy and ill adolescents. So many dramatic changes occur within the normal healthy adolescent body that substantial emphasis should be directed toward assessing adolescents' knowledge of normal growth and development. By informing adolescents of present and anticipatory physiologic changes, anxiety and confusion regarding body changes may be markedly lessened. Education can assure adolescents that the physical changes and psychological and social uncertainty associated with this time period are normal. The evolution of new relationships with family, friends, and peers often produces great uncertainty and distress, but working through this natural phenomenon with open communication can lead to close and meaningful bonds with others as adolescents mature into adulthood.

Defining Adolescence

Adolescence is a broad age range that begins with the appearance of the secondary sex characteristics at approximately 12 years of age and ends with the completion of somatic growth at about 19 years of age (Betz, Hunsberger, & Wright, 1994). However, the end of adolescence is open to debate. Some definitions of adolescence include a more comprehensive social context rather than a strict chronologic age range. These definitions mark the end of adolescence with social maturity, economic independence, and emancipation from family (Scipien, Barnard, Chard, Howe, & Phillips,

1986). Economic independence further blurs adolescent boundaries. Many individuals are well into their second decade of life before they achieve economic independence and enter into mature, responsible adulthood. Thus, from a socioeconomic perspective, adolescence may be extended by as much as five or more years beyond the completion of the other phases of growth and development.

Adolescence is further divided into the subphases of early (11–14 years of age), middle (14–17 years of age), and late adolescence (17–20 years of age). Although the primary psychosocial developmental task of adolescence is to consolidate social, sexual, and vocational identity, each subphase adds a specific, crucial component toward this developmental consolidation (Herold & Marshall, 1996). Each subphase produces specific changes. For example, adolescents learn about and respond to the rapid physiologic changes of puberty during early adolescence. During middle adolescence, a greater focus is placed on social issues whereby the establishment of peer relations and heterosexual interests assume importance. Late adolescence involves the incorporation of adult roles and the development of intimacy in relationships.

Puberty

From a physiologic perspective, puberty is the hallmark of the beginning of adolescence and encompasses sexual maturation and physical growth (Sieving & Bearinger, 1995). Females enter puberty two years earlier than males (Betz et al., 1994), with the earliest visible signs of breast changes occurring at a mean age of 11 years with a range of 9–13.5 years (Sieving & Bearinger). Among males, testicular pubertal changes are the earliest visible sign of puberty and occur between 9.5 and 14 years of age (Sieving & Bearinger). Sexual maturation rates vary tremendously among adolescents. This variation can be a source of substantial stress as adolescents seek to be similar to their peers but may be well ahead of or behind them in pubertal development.

Dramatic physical growth takes place during puberty. This accelerated growth spurt generally lasts two to three years and encompasses skeletal, muscular, and internal organ growth (Sieving & Bearinger, 1995). During puberty, skeletal mass and muscle, or lean body mass, actually doubles, as does the size of the heart, lungs, spleen, kidneys, pancreas, uterus, gonads, and phallus (Betz et al., 1994). Brain growth continues during puberty and allows for the increase in cognitive function.

During this growth period, almost every aspect of the adolescent's body is affected. Hormonal influences and bone development cause facial structures to change. Integumentary changes and problems with acne frequently are experienced. Legs lengthen dramatically, contributing to the lanky and clumsy appearance so typical during this phase. Females experience a substantial increase in body fat that creates much turmoil and difficulty for them during this period.

Theories of Adolescence

G. Stanley Hall

Numerous and varying theories of adolescence exist. G. Stanley Hall, known as the father of adolescence, was the first psychologist to formulate a theory of adolescence. The theory was based largely on biogenetics. Hall applied Charles Darwin's concept of biologic evolution and developed a psychological theory of progression whereby individuals proceed through stages of development similar to how mankind proceeded through stages of development in history. In Hall's view, physiologic change causes development, and environment is of little relevance. He proposed that the numerous physiologic changes cause psychological changes. These physiologic changes create "sturm and drang," a German phrase meaning storm and stress. Adolescence, in his view, is a transitional, turbulent stage. Hall viewed the emotional life of adolescents as an oscillation of contradictory tendencies whereby adolescents characteristically oscillate between extremes of emotions (Muuss, 1996). For example, adolescents can be moody and melancholic one moment and giddy and euphoric the next. Adolescents can exhibit mature and immature behavior. They may want to isolate themselves and later become consumed with their peer relationships. Adolescence is a time of idealism, commitment to beliefs, rebellion, passion, and expression of feelings. Behavior can range from pure egocentrism to actions that convey extreme concern for others. Unlike other theorists who claim adolescence ends earlier, Hall defined the end of adolescence as the time when full adult status is obtained (approximately 22–25 years of age) (Muuss, 1988).

Margaret Mead

Margaret Mead was a cultural anthropologist who was best known for her landmark research about adolescents that was documented in *Coming of Age in Samoa*. Mead observed that stress, turmoil, sexual frustration, and crises of growing up associated with the age group were not universal phenomena among adolescents but were very much contingent on cultural setting, child-rearing practices, and social-environmental issues (Muuss, 1988). Her research in Samoan society revealed adolescence as a smooth, tranquil, and carefree time period characterized by harmonious interactions with others (Muuss, 1988). According to Mead, the carefree adolescent behavior she observed was the result of cultural learning and socialization, not biologic determinism.

Formal Operations

Along with the rapid physiologic changes that occur with puberty, cognitive capacity also changes. According to the Piagetian stages of cognitive development, young adolescents proceed from the stage of concrete operations into the final stage of cognitive development that is known as formal operations (Muuss, 1996). Formal operational thought allows adolescents to consider all of the possible combinations of propositions and their interrelationships (Newman & Newman, 1997). The ability to review evidence using abstract thinking and hypothetical reasoning before coming to a logical conclusion characterizes this stage (Jarvis, 1996). The development of abstract thinking and logical reasoning paves the way for thinking about values and assessing family values. Adolescents in the formal operations stage can contemplate future possibilities beyond the present reality and mentally form ideals, which leads to idealism.

Derived from Piaget's theory of cognitive development, egocentrism is another important concept related to adolescence. Egocentrism is defined as the lack of differentiation between a person's own point of view and the points of view of others (Muuss, 1996). Although adolescents are beginning to conceptualize the thought processes of others, they cannot yet differentiate others' concerns from their own (Betz et al., 1994). Adolescent egocentrism is an adolescent's false belief that others are just as interested in his or her own actions, behaviors, assets, weaknesses, and appearance as the adolescent is. Thus, adolescent egocentrism characteristically involves adolescents thinking that they are the focus of interest of other people. Elkind (1967) refers to this as an "imaginary audience."

Adolescents' belief that they are the center of attention, especially among peers, contributes to their self-consciousness.

Elkind also uses the term "personal fable" in reference to adolescents' sense of indestructibility and invincibility. Adolescents' perception of their special uniqueness—the idea that no one could possibly understand them—is engendered in this personal fable. By virtue of their uniqueness, adolescents characteristically believe that nothing can harm them. This belief can be used to understand and explain adolescent risk-taking behaviors. Adolescents begin to experience the personal fable and imaginary audience in early adolescence, and they diminish in late adolescence.

Harry Stack Sullivan

Harry Stack Sullivan's interpersonal theory of development focuses on interpersonal relationships and is based largely on social psychiatry and communication. This theory emphasizes the importance of social approval and disapproval for the development of self. One of Sullivan's major contributions to personality theory was the idea that the intrapsychic component could be observed only indirectly through interpersonal interactions with others (Muuss, 1996). Instead of explaining human development in terms of biologic determinism, sexuality, or intrapsychic dynamics, Sullivan focused on the social context of human experiences. The self-system, which is a part of personality, is an important concept of this theory. The way in which significant others interact with, view, and respond to individuals shapes the self-system, which is based on reflective appraisal by these significant others (Muuss, 1988). Self—that is, the way in which individuals see themselves—is based largely on or influenced by social interactions with others. One of the important functions of the self-system is to provide satisfaction and reduce anxiety when dealing with others (Muuss, 1996). The self-system serves to maintain equilibrium and is essential to adjustment because it maintains self-respect, facilitates security, and minimizes anxiety.

Sullivan's theory has three adolescent phases: preadolescence, early adolescence, and late adolescence. Preadolescence begins with a change in social orientation whereby the need for an intense, interpersonal intimacy with a member of the same sex emerges and ends with the eruption of genital sexuality during puberty (Muuss, 1996). During early adolescence, the object of intimacy shifts from a member of the same sex to heterosexual relationships. The shifting period often involves great insecurity, fear, and wishful thinking about the desired individual (Muuss, 1996). This insecurity is both internal and external. Adolescents are clumsy in their approach toward the opposite sex and experience mental conflicts and confusion about heterosexual interests. External insecurities (e.g., communication problems, stereotypes, interpersonal difficulties) are evident in interactions (Muuss, 1988). Late adolescence is the period when adolescents can satisfy their sexual needs and are capable of mature interpersonal relationships. The distinction between early and late adolescence clearly is the achievement of sexual gratification.

Sexual activity, according to Sullivan, is necessary for the development and attainment of mature interpersonal relationships that are based on mutual respect (Muuss, 1988). To form a unified whole as an individual and proceed into adulthood, adolescents need to experiment with all aspects of the self-system (Muuss, 1988).

Although Sullivan's theory is similar to Freud's in that adolescence is viewed as the genital stage, their theories are discernibly distinct. Sullivan's theoretical underpinnings are based on social interaction and the self in relationship to others. Conversely, Freud's genital stage, or adolescence proper, is based on an intrapsychic construct (i.e., the ego) (Muuss, 1996).

Sigmund Freud

Freud, the originator of psychoanalysis, was a Viennese physician. He conceptualized that the human personality was made up of three components: id, ego, and superego. The id, or the unconscious mind, is the biologic component that is driven by instinct (sexual and aggressive drive) and seeks gratification. According to Freud, the unconscious is the dominant force of the mind, especially in psychopathologic states. The ego, or the conscious mind, is the reality-oriented function. As children grow, the ego develops with an increasing ability to satisfy both ego and id impulses in a socially acceptable manner. The superego, or conscience, represents the moral or ethical component and functions to prevent individuals from revealing instincts considered to be socially unacceptable. These three components are integrated and coalesce into a healthy personality that can interact and satisfy basic needs and desires within socially prescribed mores (Muuss, 1996).

Freud's stages of psychosexual development proceed in a sequential, predetermined fashion according to the body zones (oral, anal, phallic, and genital) that provide libidinous satisfaction for each of the specific developmental periods (Muuss, 1996). For each stage, there is conflict regarding the expression of sexual and aggressive drives. In Freud's psychoanalytic perspective, individuals experience opposing conflicts between their natural instincts, or basic drives, and their societal constraints (Papalia & Olds, 1986). Each of the stages reflects a different bodily focus where pleasure is obtained and intertwined with social interactions. Freud believed that the five psychosexual stages are universal, and individuals must proceed through these stages in order to become mature adults. Disruptions can occur in the normal process of sequential stages, which result in fixation and regression. Fixation is a developmental arrest that results from either overgratification or too little gratification during a specific psychosexual stage (Papalia & Olds). When this occurs, the individual remains at an immature level of gratification and does not proceed to higher levels (Muuss, 1996).

Freud described adolescence as the genital stage, characterized by a reawakening of the sexual drive (Jarvis, 1996). Unlike the school-age years, or latency period, when sexual drives can be repressed, adolescents now seek gratification of sexual urges. The genital stage begins at puberty with maturation of the reproductive system and production of the sex hormones (Rollins, 1995). A rapid increase in sexual tension that demands gratification marks this stage, but these sexual and aggressive biologic drives must be integrated into socially acceptable intimate relationships (Muuss, 1988). The id, ego, and superego are in conflict as adolescents struggle with id impulses, which are creating a desire for biologic gratification, and the superego, which is responsible for moral behavior. Because of this conflict, the ego is unable to balance the other two. Hence, psychological disequilibrium commonly is seen during adolescence.

One of Freud's most significant and widely recognized contributions was the identification of defense mechanisms (Muuss, 1996). Defense mechanisms assist the ego to cope with frustration, anxiety, and impulsive behavior and to reduce tension and internal conflicts (Muuss, 1988). Although Freud focused predominantly on the defense mechanism of repression, his daughter, Anna, expanded his work and comprehensively addressed the ego's defensive aspects. She described adolescents' use of intellectualization and asceticism in helping to deal with emergent sexual drives (Kaplan & Sadock, 1998).

Freud was the first to systematically consider denial as a clinical construct. He viewed all defenses as unconscious mental processes functioning as psychological barriers between the instinctual drives and the external realities of life (Levine, Rudy, & Kerns, 1994). Because denial unconsciously blocks or distorts external reality, psychoanalysts have considered it to be a pathologic response. However, Anna Freud's later work extended the construct of denial, which, in her view, was a normal childhood defense. The use of defense mechanisms increases during adolescence as a result of the rapid developmental changes taking place. Although all of the defense mechanisms distort reality, denial is an especially primitive defense that distorts reality and denies the existence of some emotionally significant part of reality (Muuss, 1996). Although Freud made highly significant contributions to the psychoanalytic approach to children and adolescents, he placed his greatest emphasis on infantile sexuality and the first five years of life, with substantially less emphasis on pubescence and adolescence (Muuss, 1988).

Erik Erikson

Erikson, in contrast to Freud, devoted special attention to the period of adolescence, and his writings popularized the term "identity" in association with adolescence (Muuss, 1996). His theory of personality development focused on predictable stages of development that are accompanied by periods of crisis in which resolution is necessary to proceed to or attain a higher stage of development. In this framework, crisis refers to a normal conflict or stressor resulting from an opposing or bipolar outcome in each of the respective stages.

Erikson believed that during each of the stages, individuals actually must experience both opposing conflicts, process the conflicts, and eventually synthesize the process. Each crisis is named for its bipolar outcome. If the conflict is resolved positively, individuals incorporate the experience into the ego, thereby facilitating healthy progression through subsequent stages of development. Being aware that a crisis never is resolved completely is important. In fact, resolution may occur during a later developmental time span, but the major accomplishment of the task is attained during the time when the conflict initially emerges and is most pronounced. In essence, individuals experience either a successful (favorable) or unsuccessful (unfavorable) outcome for each of the sequential stages. Unsuccessful resolution—when the conflict continues past its reasonable time—results in impairment of further development and may present itself in problems with adjustment, self-concept, and even psychopathologic conditions (Muuss, 1996).

Erikson's eight stages of psychosocial development are perhaps the most widely accepted and used theory, partly because of the focus on healthy personality development rather than psychopathology (Rollins, 1995). Unlike many other personality theorists whose stages of development end in adolescence or young adulthood, Erikson's eight stages of psychosocial development reflect a lifespan approach from infancy through senescence.

Erikson's fifth stage (the adolescent stage)—identity versus role confusion—corresponds to Freud's genital stage. The important task for the 12–18-year-old is establishing a sense of personal identity that is based on all of the characteristics that establish who people are and where they are going (Kaplan & Sadock, 1998). Because it occurs during the rapid physiologic changes of puberty, this developmental task is a challenging and difficult one. The process of searching for identity requires that individuals establish a meaningful self-concept based on success in attaining trust, autonomy, initiative, and industry during earlier stages. According to Erikson (1963), confusion is expected as adolescents struggle with changes in skeletal growth, libidinal drives, and the development of secondary sex characteristics. As part of this process, adolescents must develop an ego identity and accept the myriad of bodily changes and libidinal urges (Muuss, 1996). Unlike the latency period of childhood, individuals' familiarity with their body no longer is a comfort. Consideration of the future, including a growing awareness of the numerous responsibilities required during the approaching period of adulthood, also creates confusion.

Identity

To facilitate the identity process, adolescents must ask the very important questions of "Who am I?" "Where did I come from?" and "What am I to become?" Identity formation requires the assimilation of past and present with an idea about what the future might hold. Vocational choices and goals have to be considered. These ultimately will form a vocational identity, which is an important component of total identity. Multiple career choices and aspirations to glamorous but relatively unobtainable roles as rock stars, supermodels, athletes, actresses, and other celebrities create common role confusion. The difficulty for adolescents lies in their ability to narrow down and select a career that they will find satisfying and rewarding and in pursuing a career that is commensurate with their cognitive and emotional capacities. Consequently, many adolescents initially stumble with their career choices. With maturity and experimentation, they eventually choose a suitable career. Making major life decisions while standing on the shaky ground of immaturity is an immense task.

Although extremely frustrating to parents, experimentation is necessary during adolescence. As difficult as it may be, the process of experimentation teaches adolescents, and they make decisions based on their experiences.

Peer relations are the major influence on adolescent identity. While searching for a personal identity, adolescents turn to their peers for approval and respond most significantly to their reactions, both positive and negative. Identity is intrinsically connected to sameness. Erikson identified the process in which adolescents experience a period of great need for peer group recognition and involvement as psychosocial reciprocity (Muuss, 1996). During this time, adolescents become extremely preoccupied with their dress and appearance because body image is intrinsically related to identity.

During early adolescence, parents may be viewed as role models and adolescents readily accept the limitations placed on them by parental authority. However, as adolescents progress through the teenage years, role models change substantially. Parental control often is viewed as overly restrictive. Later in adolescence, teenagers rarely identify with their parents; instead, they identify with their peer group and the teen idols of the day. Varying degrees of rebellion that lead to conflicts with parents characterize adolescence. These rebellious actions against parental control and values are, in fact, quite normal and healthy because adolescents need to be autonomous and must separate from their family and parental identity to form their own unique identity. While rebelling against their parents' values, they must develop their own value system that is congruent with the mores of society. Integrating these values, they must develop their own philosophy of life from which to gauge and direct their choices and behavior (Muuss, 1996).

Moral Development

Morality is considered to be a major accomplishment of late adolescence and adulthood (Kaplan & Sadock, 1998). Morality is defined as conformity to shared standards, rights, and duties (Kaplan &

Sadock). According to Lawrence Kohlberg (1968), moral development is based on cognitive developmental theory. It consists of three levels, and each has two stages. Each level follows a predetermined sequence: preconventional, conventional, and postconventional. At the preconventional level, children conform to the rules imposed by parents and authority figures. At the conventional level, children are concerned with conformity and social order to gain approval and promote maintenance of family relationships. At the postconventional level, the last and most advanced level, children no longer approach moral dilemmas based on their own needs or the need for conformity; instead, they comply with rules based on autonomous principles of justice. Similar to Freud who felt that women were morally inferior to men, Kohlberg's theory reflects a more contemporary view of women's moral inferiority.

Carol Gilligan's *In a Different Voice* (1982) challenged Kohlberg's theory of moral development, for she maintains that Kohlberg's theory fails to consider women's concerns. Her research identified discernible differences in gender-based moral development that Kohlberg did not address. Gilligan's theory highlights gender differences. As a result of the individuation process during early childhood, women tend to remain connected and have greater sensitivity and concern for others than men. While societal expectations mandate that men use independent judgment and assertiveness, women naturally focus on the concern for the well-being of others. This creates a substantial moral dilemma for women, whether to be concerned for self or others, which is not at all addressed by Kohlberg.

Identity Crisis

By the end of adolescence, individuals have undergone all of these tremendous changes with the concomitant physical, intellectual, emotional, vocational, and societal expectations and stressors. Although an identity crisis is expected and normal during adolescence, failure to resolve this crisis is problematic. When a positive outcome is not achieved, young adults deal with negative bipolar outcome (i.e., confusion). Confusion about themselves and their place and role in the world and not knowing who they are or where they are going characterize daily adolescent life (Kaplan & Sadock, 1998). Long-term confusion often manifests in adjustment problems, poor self-concept, and self-destructive activities, thereby complicating young adulthood with serious unresolved issues.

References

Betz, C.L., Hunsberger, M.M., & Wright, S. (1994). *Family-centered nursing care of children* (2nd ed.). Philadelphia: W.B. Saunders.

Elkind, D. (1967). Egocentrism in adolescence. *Child Development, 38,* 1025–1034.

Erikson, E.H. (1963). *Childhood and society.* New York: Norton & Co.

Gilligan, C. (1982). *In a different voice.* Cambridge, MA: Harvard University Press.

Herold, E.S., & Marshall, S.K. (1996). Adolescent sexual development. In G.R. Adams, R. Montemayor, & T.P. Gullotta (Eds.), *Psychosocial development during adolescence: Progress in developmental contextualism* (pp. 62–94). Thousand Oaks, CA: Sage.

Jarvis, C. (1996). *Physical examination and health assessment* (2nd ed.). Philadelphia: W.B. Saunders.

Kaplan, H.I., & Sadock, B.J. (1998). *Kaplan & Sadock's synopsis of psychiatry: Behavioral sciences/clinical psychiatry* (8th ed.). Baltimore: Williams & Wilkins.

Kohlberg, L. (1968). Moral development. In D.L. Sills (Ed.), *International encyclopedia of the social sciences* (vol. 10) (pp. 483–494). New York: MacMillan.

Levine, J., Rudy, T., & Kerns, R. (1994). A two-factor model of denial of illness: A confirmatory factor analysis. *Journal of Psychosomatic Research, 38,* 99–110.

Muuss, R. (1988). *Theories of adolescence* (5th ed.) New York: Random House.

Muuss, R. (1996). *Theories of adolescence* (6th ed.). New York: McGraw-Hill.

Newman, P., & Newman, B.M. (1997). *Childhood and adolescence.* New York: Brooks/Cole Publishing.

Papalia, D., & Olds, S. (1986). *Human development* (3rd ed.). New York: McGraw-Hill.

Rollins, J. (1995). Growth and development in children. In D. Wong (Ed.), *Whaley & Wong's nursing care of infants and children* (5th ed.) (pp. 106–154). St. Louis: Mosby.

Scipien, G.M., Barnard, M.U., Chard, M.A., Howe, J., & Phillips, P.J. (1986). *Comprehensive pediatric nursing* (3rd ed.). New York: McGraw-Hill.

Sieving, R., & Bearinger, L. (1995). Health promotion of the adolescent and family. In D. Wong (Ed.), *Whaley & Wong's nursing care of infants and children* (5th ed.) (pp. 825–861). St. Louis: Mosby.

CHAPTER 2.

Psychosocial Issues of Seriously Ill Adolescents

Kathleen L. Neville, PhD, RN

Introduction

The rapid changes of puberty, including all of the physiologic, cognitive, social, and emotional factors, are capable of creating tremendous havoc and turmoil for adolescents transitioning toward adulthood. Although this course varies dramatically among healthy adolescents, the onset of a serious and potentially life-threatening illness undoubtedly alters the sequence and timing of reaching these important development stages. How cancer affects adolescent development—whether it speeds up, slows down, or redirects development—is an important question (Hinds, 1997).

As advances in biomedical science and technology have dramatically and steadily improved survival rates throughout the last 30 years, substantial research has been conducted regarding the psychosocial functioning of children with cancer. Since the 1960s, more than 200 investigations about the psychosocial aspects of adjustment, coping, or adaptation to pediatric cancer have been conducted (Kupst, 1994). Although much emphasis has been placed on children's reactions to serious illness and pediatric cancer, far less attention has been given to the experience of illness during adolescence. This may be partly because of the scope of pediatrics—the period from infancy through adolescence. Although adolescent care is subsumed under the broad umbrella of child care and pediatrics, adolescence is a unique developmental time span. Adolescents are beyond childhood, but they are not yet adults. Additionally, adolescents have special needs and concerns that often differ from the physical and psychosocial problems of adults or younger children with cancer (Cohen & Klopovich, 1986).

Psychosocial Research Issues

In recent years, researchers have focused their attention on the need to conduct more rigorous studies because much of the earlier research was anecdotal and descriptive and lacked theoretical foundation or hypothesis testing (Kupst, 1994). Although clinical observations support the existence of psychological distress in children and adolescents with cancer, empirical documentation during crisis points is needed (Rait & Holland, 1986).

Kupst described some basic assumptions that have guided psychological research regarding pediatric cancer. Many researchers have used and continue to use a pathology-oriented model that identifies children with cancer as a potentially at-risk population for psychological difficulties. With this type of model, personality inventories commonly are used and the psychological problems of anxiety, depression, hostility, and family dysfunction frequently are assessed. Studies also have been conducted using a normative-based model. With a normative-based model, families faced with cancer are viewed as normal people who are confronted with tremendous life stressors. In these studies, the process of coping with the stressful events of the illness is emphasized.

Earlier studies focused on the parents, particularly mothers' responses to the illness. But, in recent years, the children have become a focus of research. Additionally, the important role of fathers, siblings, the extended family, and even the community has been recognized. The availability of social networks and social support has been studied largely as an important factor in the psychological adjustment process. Much of the research has been cross-sectional in that the phenomena of interest at one specific time has been investigated. Examples of cross-sectional studies include the time periods of the crisis of diagnosis, the waiting period, the dying phase, and long-term survivorship. Longitudinal studies, which capture the dynamic processes of living with and through the cancer experience, reveal the important changes experienced throughout time. This type of study is appearing more frequently in the literature and provides important advances in knowledge.

Scientific advances in pediatric cancer have yielded incredible improvements in long-term survival of children and adolescents with cancer. Substantial theoretical knowledge about coping styles and psychosocial adjustment to cancer has provided healthcare professionals with effective assessment tools and intervention strategies to assist adolescents and their families in dealing with the cancer experience. Research has identified the population most at risk for psychological difficulties when faced with adolescent cancer. These risk factors include lack of emotional support, severe physical problems, limited financial resources, compromised coping abilities, and increased stressors.

Cancer's Effect on Adolescence

Adolescents with cancer experience many illness-related stressors in addition to the normal physical and psychosocial stressors that are associated with this age period (Baum & Baum, 1990). At a time in life when adolescents are focusing on the achievement of the most fundamental and important task of this age period—consolidating their identity—illness interferes dramatically with all aspects of it.

The need to conform to peers and be alike in appearance, style, actions, and dress characterizes adolescence. For adolescents, being the same as others is vitally important to developing self-concept. An illness such as cancer and, specifically, cancer treatment, with its potential to alter appearance, can severely hinder or permanently scar the formation of identity. Adolescents are normally quite anxious about the numerous body changes (e.g., size, shape, secondary sex characteristics). The host of treatment-related side effects (e.g., alopecia, edema, body weight changes, disfiguring surgery) that are superimposed on normal bodily concerns can result in feelings of worthlessness and diminished self-concept (Carr-Gregg & White, 1987). Adolescence is an especially difficult time to be viewed as different from peers. Many adolescents respond to this major stressor by withdrawing from social interactions that normally facilitate psychosocial development (Vessey & Swanson, 1996).

Even among healthy adolescents, achieving autonomy and independence is seldom smooth and effortless. It frequently involves much conflict, stress, loss, and sorrow as adolescents disengage from their parents and shift toward a peer group. However, when adolescents are diagnosed with cancer, they are forced to rely on parents for major treatment decisions, provision of care, and intense support. Children's and adolescents' need for parental and family support is perhaps greatest during illness. Despite significant social changes, the family remains the major source of social support for adolescents with cancer and fills a void related to peer support (Neville, 1998; Stovall & Peacock, 1984; Tebbi, Stern, Boyle, Mettlin, & Mindell, 1985). During interviews with survivors of adolescent cancer (see Chapter 5), participants related their need for the intense support and constant devotion of their parents and significant others.

The whole hospital experience (e.g., rules, procedures, time demands, fixed schedules, noise levels, waiting time, delays, follow-up appointments) also thwarts autonomy, fosters dependence, and promotes a sense of helplessness.

At a time when healthy adolescents begin thinking about their future and long-term plans, adolescents with a life-threatening illness shift their focus to the present. Adolescents with cancer are confronted with ambiguity and uncertainty regarding their future, including the awareness of a potentially limited life expectancy. After the initial diagnostic period, also known as the existential plight in cancer, adolescents begin rethinking their future aspirations and consider changes in premorbid hopes and dreams regarding education, career, marriage, family, and reproductive issues. Although long-term survivorship is increasingly a realistic outcome, many adolescents with cancer will face varying degrees of impairment, permanent disability, or death. For some unfortunate adolescents, illness prevents the completion of developmental tasks.

Psychological Distress Among Adolescents With Cancer

Despite all of the significant scientific advances, cancer is still the leading cause of nonaccidental and nonsuicide adolescent deaths. Because of this, a cancer diagnosis is one of the most frightening to receive and understandably is associated with tremendous psychological distress (Derogatis et al., 1983; Wool & Goldberg, 1986). Anxiety, depression, and hostility often are signs of psychological distress (Zevon, Tebbi, & Stern, 1987). The diagnosis and treatment phases of cancer are difficult times for adolescents and family members (Rait & Holland, 1986). Many parents report the period of diagnosis as "the hardest blow they had to bear throughout the course of the illness" (Binger et al., 1969, p. 415). Weisman and Worden (1976–77) recognized the importance of this period, which they described as "the existential plight in cancer." It refers to the experience of any severe emotional stress beginning with the actual diagnosis and early treatment and extending approximately 100 days after. Almost all patients with cancer experience this highly significant yet poorly recognized time of vulnerability. Psychological distress is a frequent sequel to a cancer diagnosis (Ganz, 1988). For example, estimates of the prevalence of psychological distress among adult patients with cancer cover a wide range. Derogatis (1986) found a range of 22%–74%, and Craig and Abeloff (1974) reported a prevalence rate of up to 90%. The literature has not clearly defined psychological distress, and it often is used interchangeably with emotional, mental, symptom, and psychosocial distress. The concept of psychological distress has been used in operational definitions of psychosocial adjustment, psychological functioning, and adaptation in which psychological distress signals adjustment problems or difficulty in adaptation. Adaptation is defined as "biopsychosocial behavior occurring within a person's individually defined range of usual behavior" (Mishel, 1988b, p. 232).

The prevalence of psychological distress in adolescents with cancer is similar to that of adults with cancer (Rait & Holland, 1986). Past researchers assumed that all adolescents would exhibit some form of psychological disturbance (Lowenberg, 1970; Moore, Holton, & Martin, 1969). More recent researchers, however, address distress as a frequent nonpathologic sequel to cancer (Blotcky & Cohen, 1985) and find that adolescents with cancer are relatively well-adjusted (Neville, 1996; Zevon et al., 1987).

In a classic study of family reactions to cancer, Binger et al. (1969) interviewed 20 parents of children with leukemia about the impact of cancer on their lives. The majority of parents, siblings, and patients exhibited "symptoms and feelings of physical distress, depression, inability to function, hostility and anger" (Binger et al., p. 415). Although these symptoms represent normal responses, this study described them as signs of maladjustment. This analysis may reflect past thinking in which a cancer diagnosis was equated with inevitable demise.

In a study of the psychological effects of illness during adolescence, Kellerman, Zeltzer, Ellenberg, Dash, and Rigler (1980) compared a sample of adolescents with leukemia, cancerous tumors, cystic fibrosis, diabetes, cardiac disease, renal failure, and rheumatologic disorders to a control group of healthy adolescents using the State-Trait Anxiety Inventory (Speilberger, Gorsuch, & Lushene, 1970), the Rosenberg Scale of Self-Esteem (Rosenberg, 1965), and the Health Locus of Control Scale (Wallston, Wallston, Kaplan, & Maides, 1976). Significant differences in locus of control were identified among the subjects. Adolescents with cancer perceived significantly less control than adolescents with diabetes. No relationships existed among visible signs of the illness, severity and course of the illness, age, number of hospitalizations, and psychological adjustment. Chronically ill adolescents whose physicians rated their prognosis as stable were less anxious than those who were rated as improving, deteriorating, or uncertain. A weak but significant inverse relationship was noted between time since diagnosis and level of anxiety as well as between time since diagnosis and locus of control. Adolescents with more recent diagnoses exhibited greater anxiety and perceived less control of their health.

In a follow-up study using the same subjects, Zeltzer, Kellerman, Ellenberg, Dash, and Rigler (1980) investigated the psychological impact of illness using a self-designed, 18-item tool that addressed adolescent concerns. Impact-of-illness scores did not differ significantly between the chronically ill group and the healthy group, as healthy adolescents reported the impact of minor illnesses such as asthma, colds, allergies, and nosebleeds. Adolescents with cancer reported that treatments caused the most distress. Cancer affected body image and disrupted schooling and family relations more than any other illness. Many adolescents reported that their illness disrupted their lives and their relationships with peers, parents, and siblings.

Psychological distress was investigated in a study of 24 inpatient and 23 outpatient adolescents with different cancers (Zevon et al., 1987). Psychological distress was measured using the Symptom Checklist 90-Revised (SCL-90-R) (Derogatis, 1977). Researchers noted a generalized distress reaction from all adolescents. Inpatient males had consistently elevated scales on all dimensions of the SCL-90-R. Researchers noted a less uniform pattern of symptom dimensions among outpatients, with males reaching higher levels of anxiety and interpersonal sensitivity. A sense of social isolation was common to male and female outpatients. Inpatients had significantly higher anxiety levels, somatization, and positive symptom index. Overall findings suggested that adolescents were relatively well-adjusted and had only mild distress reactions.

The Brief Symptom Inventory (BSI) (Derogatis & Spencer, 1982), a shortened version of the SCL-90-R, has been used to study psychological distress among adolescents. The BSI is a 53-item measure, with each item rated for psychological distress using a 5-point Likert scale (0 = not at all to

4 = extreme) on nine symptom dimensions. The nine symptom dimensions are (a) anxiety (manifested by restlessness, nervousness, tension, free-floating anxiety, and panic), (b) depression (a broad range of clinical symptoms including loss of energy, lack of interest in previous activities, and dysphoric affect and mood), (c) hostility (thoughts, feelings, and actions characterized by irritability, annoyance, arguments, temper outbursts, and an urge to break things), (d) interpersonal sensitivity (feelings of personal inadequacy and inferiority), (e) obsessive-compulsive thoughts and actions (unwanted and unremitting), (f) paranoid ideation (mode of thinking involving a high degree of projection and suspiciousness), (g) phobic anxiety (a fear response to moving away from familiar and safe surroundings), (h) psychoticism (social alienation), and (i) somatization (arising from the perception of bodily dysfunction) (Derogatis & Melisaratos, 1983). In addition, the BSI contains four items that refer to poor appetite, difficulty falling asleep, thoughts of death or dying, and feelings of guilt.

In another study of psychological distress in adolescents with cancer, Baider and Kaplan De-Nour (1989) used the BSI to examine the effect of a group therapy program on 16 adolescents and young adults between 15 and 25 years of age who were living in Israel. The BSI first was administered to all 16 adolescents and then was repeated three months later with eight in the group who were participating in a weekly dynamic support group. The parents of the adolescents involved in the support group also completed the BSI. Adolescents who were attending the support group had been diagnosed within 18 months; the remaining eight, who had declined the group activity, had been diagnosed within the past 6 months. No significant differences in psychological distress were noted between the two groups. Age and education did not affect psychological distress. Adolescents in the therapy group who had a longer duration of illness experienced greater distress. Findings revealed that all adolescents had mild psychological distress with the highest subscale of anxiety. All parents reported psychological distress. An analysis of the group process revealed an initial stage in which members described their diagnoses, reactions, and bodily experiences followed by dialogue that emphasized normality and health. Normal adolescent concerns (e.g., peer relationships, romance, parents, military service, future educational plans) were the focus of discussion. No reference was made to the interference or limitations from cancer. Therapists' attempts to address the realistic issues of cancer were denied and dismissed. Contrary to Kellerman et al.'s (1980) findings that recently diagnosed adolescents were more anxious and perceived less control, Baider and Kaplan De-Nour found that newly diagnosed adolescents or adolescents undergoing active cancer treatment used more denial.

Blackmore (1988) conducted a study to compare psychological status of males with testicular cancer who had undergone a unilateral orchidectomy to men who had undergone orchidectomy for nonmalignant conditions and a control group of men who were visiting their physician for nontesticular health problems. Ages ranged from 18–45 years. Psychological distress was determined by obtaining the Positive Symptom Distress Index, an intensity measure of the BSI (Derogatis & Spencer, 1982). Even after controlling for age, marital status, and social class, findings revealed no significant differences in psychological distress among the three groups.

Using a developmental framework in a descriptive, longitudinal study, Weekes (1989) investigated how adolescents cope with pain related to cancer treatment. Adolescents reported cancer treatments as physically, mentally, and psychologically painful. However, most adolescents reported believing that they had the ability to cope with and even lessen the treatment-related pain. Confrontative strategies (e.g., information seeking, anticipatory problem solving, attempts to control) were predominately used along with the mental-cognitive strategy of not thinking about the treatments.

The BSI also was used in a study to determine the prevalence of psychological distress among adolescents who had been diagnosed with cancer within the past 100 days (Neville, 1993, 1996). No significant differences in psychological distress were found between the healthy and ill groups when compared to normative data of healthy adolescents. Length of time was examined and trichotomized into the first 4 weeks after diagnosis, 8 weeks after diagnosis, and 12 weeks after diagnosis. Although not statistically significant, a pattern was revealed between length of time and psychological distress: distress increased from a mean of 0.69 at 4 weeks after diagnosis to 0.74 at 8 weeks after diagnosis to 0.85 at 14 weeks after diagnosis. In this study, researchers found that psychological distress may increase throughout time. Adolescent diseases then were categorized into five groups: leukemia, bone tumors, lymphoma, testicular, and other cancers (e.g., brain, ovarian, thyroid, melanoma, soft tissue, orbital). Upon examination of the two subscales, somatization and anxiety, significant differences were found. Post-hoc comparisons using the Scheffe tests to determine specifically which groups were different revealed that adolescents with leukemia had significantly higher somatization and anxiety scores than adolescents with other types of cancer (Neville, 1993, 1996). However, the data should be interpreted cautiously because the items on the somatization scale tap many common side effects of treatment (e.g., nausea, vomiting, dizziness, chest pain, numbness in any part of the body). Speculative reasons for these findings may be related to the frequency of bone marrow aspirations and spinal taps commonly performed after diagnosis and the awareness of a long maintenance treatment plan. Consultations with oncology nurse clinicians and oncologists provided additional speculation that children and adolescents tend to view leukemia as a systemic disease. In contrast, children and adolescents view malignancies such as bone tumors as localized diseases. Additionally, the oncology professionals speculated that when extensive surgery is involved (as in bone tumors), the focus shifts during the first three months from the illness to the surgical experience. The findings from this study suggest that additional studies to investigate differences among the various types of adolescent cancers are warranted.

In this same study, gender also was investigated to determine whether any significant differences existed in psychological distress between adolescent males and females recently diagnosed with cancer. Findings revealed no differences between males and females, which is contrary to the findings of Zevon et al. (1987), who found consistently elevated psychological distress scores among male inpatients who had been diagnosed with cancer.

Assessing the impact of cancer on the psychosocial functioning of adolescents is a complicated issue (Stern, Norman, & Zevon, 1993). Adolescents' appraisal of the stressful event and factors associated with psychological adjustment are crucial aspects of their psychological response to cancer. Some of the factors identified in the literature are uncertainty, use of denial or adaptive denial, and social support.

Uncertainty in Illness

Florence Nightingale (1992) described the way that uncertainty negatively affects patients: "Apprehension, uncertainty, waiting, expectation, and fear of surprise do a patient more harm than any exertion. Remember, he is face to face with the enemy all the time, internally wrestling with him, having long imaginary conversations with him" (p. 22).

Koocher and O'Malley (1981) described uncertainty in pediatric cancer as the "Damocles syndrome," which is named for a courtier in ancient Syracuse whose king invited him to a lavish banquet but arranged his seat directly below a sword suspended by a single thread. Although progress in medical science has created realistic hopes for survival, the life of any child or adolescent with cancer is in peril.

Uncertainty has been identified as the most striking feature of childhood cancer (Van Dongen-Melman, Pruyn, Van Zanen, & Sanders-Woudstra, 1986) and a major concern of adolescents with cancer (Bearison & Pacifici, 1984; Brunnquell & Hall, 1982). During interviews with families of children with cancer, Clarke-Steffen (1993) found that families reported the worst part of the experience as the "waiting and not knowing" while their child was being diagnosed.

Uncertainty has been defined in the broad context of risk, choice, probability, and decision making. Parsons (1980) stated that "exposure to uncertainty is perhaps the most negative aspect of human life and action as distinguished from lower forms of living systems" (p. 145). Mishel (1981a) developed a nursing model of uncertainty in illness to investigate the role of uncertainty as a perceptual variable that influences appraisal of events related to hospitalization, illness, and treatment. This model later developed into a theory of uncertainty in illness based on the theories of cognitive appraisal, illness-related events, stress and coping, information processing, and chaos. Uncertainty in illness occurs when individuals are unable to recognize or classify stimuli and form a cognitive schema, or a subjective evaluation of the meaning of illness-related events. Mishel and Braden (1988) concisely defined uncertainty as "the inability to determine the meaning of events, assign definite values to objects and events, or accurately predict outcomes" (p. 98).

Uncertainty in illness related to symptoms, diagnosis, prognosis, treatments, and relationships with caregivers occurs when stimuli are ambiguous (Christman et al., 1988). When illness-related events are not distinct, available, specific, or familiar (Mishel, 1981b), they cannot be categorized adequately and uncertainty ensues (Budner, 1962).

Mishel's (1988a) uncertainty in illness theory addresses three components: the antecedents of uncertainty, impaired cognitive appraisal, and coping with uncertainty in illness. The primary antecedent, or stimulus frame, is the perceived stimuli regarding the pattern of symptoms, familiarity with events, and congruence between expected and experienced illness-related events (Mishel, 1988b). Patients use the stimulus frame to structure a cognitive schema and reduce uncertainty (Mishel, 1988b; Mishel & Braden, 1988). Two additional antecedent variables, cognitive capacity and structure providers, affect the stimulus frame. Cognitive capacity may become impaired during illness and result in difficulty perceiving symptom patterns and event familiarity and congruence. Structure providers are the resources that are available to assist individuals in interpreting the stimulus frame, and they consist of individuals' social support, credible authority, and educational level. Structure providers can reduce uncertainty directly by interpreting the illness-related events or indirectly by providing assistance in interpreting the stimulus frame (Mishel & Braden, 1988).

When uncertainty is appraised as a danger and a harmful outcome is anticipated, coping efforts are used to reduce uncertainty (Mishel, 1988b). If coping efforts are effective, adaptation occurs. Difficulty in adaptation is congruent with psychological distress, poor psychosocial adjustment, and family adjustment problems (Koocher & O'Malley, 1981).

Uncertainty about outcomes, meanings, and consequences of events is important to individuals facing an illness. Managing the uncertainty in illness and treatment is a vital task in adapting to those events (Mishel, 1988b). In summary, uncertainty is a cognitive state that is created when individuals cannot adequately categorize or structure events because of lack of sufficient cues. Uncertainty results in an inability to determine the meaning of illness-related events (Mishel, 1988b).

For individuals to form a cognitive schema (e.g., a subjective evaluation of meaning of illness-related events), they must be able to classify and recognize events. Stimuli must be clear, consistent, familiar, limited in number, and clear in boundaries (Mishel, 1988a). For newly diagnosed patients with cancer, events occurring during hospitalization and treatment seldom meet these criteria. Symptoms generally are ambiguous and may be quite novel to those newly diagnosed. Seeking care in a large treatment center, meeting numerous healthcare specialists, initiating radiation or chemotherapy treatments, and undergoing surgery are new experiences that can overload patients with unfamiliar cues. When events cannot be categorized adequately, uncertainty is then experienced (Budner, 1962). Events appraised as uncertain are foreboding or ominous and potentiate the dangers of a life-threatening illness.

Cohen and Martinson (1988) conducted a longitudinal study using a semi-structured interview guide with a sample of 10 families in which a child had been diagnosed with cancer. At the time of diagnosis, children's ages ranged from four months to 11.7 years. Children in five of these families survived. All families identified uncertainty as a major stress-producing event for them. In another report using intensive interviews with the same sample, Martinson and Cohen (1988) found that when physicians discussed prognoses in terms of probabilities, family members had wide variations of interpretations of risks and probabilities. Many parents reported difficulty in comprehending information. Uncertainty regarding the children's current status and prognoses was a major source of stress. Researchers found a similar pattern in an investigation of 60 British families of children with leukemia (Comaroff & Maguire, 1981) who also discussed the need to meet with other families dealing with the same affliction to ease their sense of isolation.

Cohen (1993) used the grounded theory approach to analyze data from four sources to describe how families live under conditions of sustained uncertainty when a child has a life-threatening, chronic illness. The sources were a cross-sectional sample of parents of 21 children with life-threatening illnesses, data from a five-year longitudinal study (Martinson & Cohen, 1988), published biographical accounts of parents of children with life-threatening diseases, and an extensive review of the literature about uncertainty. Children in this study had hemophilia, cancer, congenital heart disease, cystic fibrosis, and Lowe's syndrome. Findings revealed that at the time of diagnosis, parents pass from a stable preillness world to one that has been shattered. The diagnosis is an assault on normalcy and disrupts the natural order of family life and relationships. Cohen reported that variation in intensity of uncertainty at diagnosis is minimal but that uncertainty fluctuates in wave-like patterns, with peaks of intensity and tolerable background levels, during periods of remission or disease control.

To manage uncertainty, parents developed strategies to manipulate the known, unknown, and unknowable. Parents focused on the present because future plans were too frightening to consider. Potentially stressful social interactions were managed, and disclosure decisions about their children's illness were made. Strategies to manage awareness of their children's disease included deliberate efforts to block or avoid thinking about the illness. Parents managed knowledge about the disease by limiting, modifying, extracting, and discounting information from healthcare professionals, depending on whether they wanted to maintain, dispel, or create uncertainty.

Levenson, Pfefferbaum, Copeland, and Silberberg (1982) investigated the information preferences of adolescents with cancer. Using a self-designed questionnaire with adolescents with cancer between the ages of 11 and 20, the researchers found that newly diagnosed patients were less likely to want additional information about their illness than adolescents who had been undergoing treatment longer. Furthermore, adolescents with an initial diagnosis and those who were not in remission engaged in defensive processes of filtering information.

Uncertainty has a direct effect on psychological distress, with a strong positive relationship noted among adolescents recently diagnosed with cancer (Neville, 1996). In this study, uncertainty about illness was a significant predictor of psychological distress. Although the cure rate has improved dramatically among adolescents with cancer, fear of death still accounts for much of the distress.

Gender Issues of Uncertainty

In relation to gender, significant differences in perceived levels of uncertainty have been found among adolescents with cancer (Neville, 1993, 1996). Although uncertainty was a significant predictor of psychological distress in males and females, separate gender-based studies revealed that uncertainty in females was a much stronger predictor of psychological distress. A possible explanation of this finding may relate to gender differences in the thinking process. Females use more connected knowledge, and males use more separate knowledge (Belenky, Clinchy, Goldberger, & Tarule, 1986). When using connected knowledge, individuals incorporate the way other people think and use a different lens to examine their views. When using separate knowledge, individuals follow rules and examine issues from a pragmatic, strategic point of view without consideration of feelings and personal beliefs. The possible use of separate knowledge by adolescent males in this study may have narrowed their focus of thinking regarding personal feelings about the uncertain aspects of cancer.

Communication Patterns of Childhood and Adolescent Illness

Inhibited or protective communication between parents and adolescents who are faced with cancer is not unusual. Bluebond-Langner (1978) observed younger children with leukemia and found that children avoid open discussions with parents to protect them from their own personal knowledge about dying. Beginning with the suspicion of a life-threatening illness, children and parents interact in a pattern of mutual pretense in which children conceal awareness of their prognosis and avoid discussions of death with parents (Bluebond-Langner). Martinson (1976) found similar results in a descriptive research program of home care for eight terminally ill children and adolescents. Parents avoided the subject of death, and children and adolescents subsequently ceased seeking information. In her work with dying children, Martinson found that children expressed a preference for open communication rather than a protected communication style of secrecy. Neville (1993) found a protective tendency in parents and, especially, adolescents, who try to offer support to parents. An 18-year-old male who recently had been diagnosed with testicular cancer described an example of this. "I hear my mother on the phone. She is so upset. She gets me crazy, so I try to make it easy for her."

Evolution of Uncertainty in Illness

Mishel (1990) reconceptualized her theory regarding the appraisal of uncertainty in illness. Substantial support exists in the pediatric cancer literature for the appraisal of uncertainty to be viewed as an aversive event at the time of diagnosis (Cohen, 1993; Cohen and Martinson, 1988;

Koocher, 1985). Although evidence supported that uncertainty in adolescents with cancer is a negative event associated with psychological distress (Neville, 1996, 1998), it also suggests that acceptance or tolerance for long-standing, chronic uncertainty may develop throughout time. Mishel (1990) theorized that the initial appraisal of uncertainty as a danger may evolve into an appraisal of uncertainty as an opportunity. As the uncertainty increases, it can exceed one's tolerance level, and the individual must learn to live with and accept living with uncertainty. This long-standing uncertainty shifts the individual from one perspective of life to a new, higher order of life. This new view of life allows the evaluation of uncertainty to be changed from an aversive event to a positive experience. Examples of this new orientation to life among people with cancer may be evidenced by the reevaluation of the fragility and impermanence in life (Mishel, 1990). One adolescent male who was undergoing induction chemotherapy commented to the researcher, "Since I've been sick, things are different. I know what is important and what is not."

Additional studies to examine the evolution of uncertainty in illness among adolescents with cancer are warranted to identify and describe what changes occur throughout time. Comaroff and Maguire (1981) described a common approach that healthcare professionals use when presenting a cancer diagnosis and treatment to children and their families. To redirect focus from long-term and existential issues, a "let's take it day to day" approach commonly is employed. Adolescents and their families learn very early during the cancer experience that relatively few certainties exist, and a newer, more complex attitude toward life evolves (Comaroff & Maguire). Although uncertainty during the early stages of illness creates fluctuation and disruption, it later becomes the foundation for constructing a new order (Mishel, 1990). Comments from a 22-year-old male one month prior to his death support this premise. When the researcher asked how he was doing, he responded, "I'm doing OK. I worry about today, getting here on time, getting chemo, and going home. I can't worry about tomorrow."

Adaptive Denial

As a defense mechanism, denial generally is conceptualized as the unconscious disavowal of an external or internal threat. Wool and Goldberg (1986) identified the importance of distinguishing among suppression, avoidance, and denial, all of which can present similarly but have clinical distinctions. Suppression is an unconscious or semiconscious process in which the defense is directed toward an intrapsychic event such as conflict or impulse. Denial is also an unconscious process that is focused against an external or internal threat in the form of an intolerable idea (Wool & Goldberg). Avoidance, on the other hand, is a knowledgeable effort to block any situations or circumstances that bring stressful information to the forefront. When using avoidance, people may be fully aware of a life-threatening illness but may attempt to deflect the conversation away from it. Signs and symptoms of anxiety and depression are often present with avoidance but absent with denial.

Denial and Childhood Cancer

In a long-term follow-up study of survivors of childhood cancer, Koocher and O'Malley (1981) reported that children react to the stress of cancer by experiencing high anxiety and other psychological adjustment problems as a result of being preoccupied with the fear that the cancer will return; believing they are immune to cancer as a result of the treatment; and not thinking about the cancer. Other researchers found that adolescents with cancer tend to function by attending to daily tasks (e.g., school events, social activities with peers, academic work) (Zeltzer, LeBaron, & Zeltzer, 1984). Koocher (1985) reported that adolescents who believe they are immune to cancer and those who do not think about it are using adaptive denial to cope with the uncertainty about the cancer. Adaptive denial is a strategy that calls for a positive, optimistic outlook on life instead of concentrating on the illness (Weekes, 1989). Martinson (1976) found that adolescent anxiety about death frequently is masked by "airs of bravado." Risk-taking behavior and jokes about death and dying are common among adolescents and are attempts to support their belief that they are at least invincible and possibly even immortal.

Verbal statements revealed examples of the use of adaptive denial by adolescents who had been diagnosed with cancer (Neville, 1993). While participating in a brief interview, one 20-year-old male with advanced testicular cancer became visibly upset when describing his liver and pulmonary metastases to the researcher. In response to a question on the Mishel Uncertainty in Illness Scale (MUIS) (Mishel & Epstein, 1990), he looked at his father and said, "Dad, this question about the seriousness of my disease has been determined. I don't think my disease is serious at all." The father's facial expression revealed bewilderment and confusion. He later was informed that adolescents normally use adaptive denial, which provides an important protective function. An 18-year-old male who maintained a nonchalant, carefree conversation about the upcoming prom while undergoing his first chemotherapy treatment is an example of how adolescents attempt to normalize their lives. Other adolescents with cancer spoke of future events (e.g., getting engaged, making plans to get married in the next few years). Although these plans were possible for many of these adolescents, they did not seem probable for some. Because of the seriousness of their disease, these "plans" may have more accurately represented adolescent hopes, dreams, and fantasies. Many adolescents demonstrated adaptive denial by expressing the strong belief that everything would turn out fine. As described in Chapter 1, the personal fable is a mental construction or story that may not be true but enables adolescents to go about everyday living without worrying about real dangers (Elkind, 1985). Along with the benefit of the personal fable, Elkind identified the negative effect of denial, which contributes to noncompliance to medical regimens.

Additionally, the literature supports that adolescents with life-threatening illnesses do not inevitably manifest psychopathological symptoms but are likely to manifest distress in one or more areas of functioning throughout the course of an illness (Kellerman et al., 1980; Zeltzer et al., 1980). Other signs of distress may be exhibited through efforts to gain a sense of control (e.g., noncompliant behavior), anxiety manifested as school phobia, separation anxiety, and increased somatic complaints (Rait & Holland, 1986).

The Multidimensional Concept of Social Support

Interest in the concept of social support has increased dramatically among the health-related disciplines throughout the past 20 years. Researchers have examined the role of social support in disease prevention, treatment, and rehabilitation and general health and well-being. Considerable amounts of research have examined whether the positive relationship between support and health occurs because support enhances health regardless of stress (known as the direct effect) or because support protects people from the harmful negative effects of stress (known as the buffering effect).

A confusing array of conceptualizations and operational measures of social support exists. Classic theorists have provided a wide range of definitions. Weiss (1974) defined social support as "the perception of relational provisions in the form of attachment, social integration, opportunity for nurturance, sense of reliable alliance, and the availability of guidance" (pp. 23–24). Cobb (1976) defined social support as "information leading the subject to believe that he is cared for and loved, esteemed, and a member of a network of mutual obligations" (p. 300). Caplan (1974) focused on the importance of feedback and reciprocity.

Varying perspectives of social support exist. Support has been conceptualized in terms of structure in interpersonal relationships. From this perspective, the existence of and interconnections between social ties are examined. Viewing support in terms of function is another perspective. From this perspective, interpersonal relations are assessed for their ability to provide affection, convey a sense of belonging, and provide material aid. The terms "expressive properties" and "instrumental properties" are used to explain social support. Expressive properties also are known as emotional and affective properties, referring to activities that convey acceptance and understanding. Instrumental properties are the tangible component (e.g., material aid, transportation, information, guidance).

Perceived, available, and received social support also are distinguishable. Although the presence of support may be expressed, it cannot be used unless it is perceived to be available (Bruhn & Philips, 1984). Most social support measures are brief, self-administered scales that are designed to assess the perception of social support (Krishnasamy, 1996). However, few of the existing scales actually measure negative social support. The measurement and identification of the negative impact of social interactions can add valuable insight to this expansive body of knowledge.

The Role of Social Support for Healthy Adolescents

Investigators have hypothesized that social support may help to buffer the effects of adverse life events on psychological health states. In a study of healthy adolescents, Aro, Hanninen, and Paronen (1989) examined the role of perceived social support in mediating the impact of adverse life events on psychosomatic symptoms. Lack of friends was associated with an increase in psychosomatic symptoms among boys and a change in symptoms among girls. Adolescents who reported a poor relationship with one or both of their parents and had experienced identified life events (e.g., change of residence, death of a grandparent, increased conflict between parents, losing a pet, birth of a sibling) had the highest psychosomatic symptoms.

Burke and Weir (1978) compared adolescent gender differences in life stress, social support received from peers and parents, and emotional well-being in healthy adolescents 13–20 years of age. Females experienced increased anxiety and tension, depression, and decreased mental and physical well-being. Females, however, discussed problems with peers more than males and reported greater satisfaction with help from peers. Males reportedly perceived less support than females. This is congruent with Ostrov, Offer, and Howard's (1989) findings from their normative study of gender differences in adolescent symptomatology among high school students that found greater psychological distress among females.

The Role of Social Support in Illness

Wortman and Dunkel-Schetter (1979) found that patients with cancer have an increased need for social support related to their uncertainty and fears associated with the diagnosis. Wortman (1984) found that patients with cancer experience difficulty in obtaining adequate support. Although many patients with cancer want to discuss their disease, family members and friends often feel threatened and anxious, which results in strained and uncomfortable interactions (Wortman; Wortman & Dunkel-Schetter).

Social support has been identified as an important multidimensional concept in determining how people adapt to cancer. Tebbi et al. (1985) examined the role of perceived social support in adaptation to cancer for adolescents who had undergone a limb amputation. Most of the participants (78%) reported that parents were the most supportive and filled a void related to lack of peer support. Less than 50% considered their friends to be helpful, 34% perceived their friends as scared and avoiding them, and 46% felt friends avoided talking about their problems. Of 27 adolescents, 17 reported adequate social support.

In a comparative study of self-image and perceived support between adolescents with cancer and healthy adolescents, Stern, Norman, and Zevon (1993) found that adolescents with cancer essentially were well-adjusted. Using the Offer Self-Image Questionnaire (Offer, Ostrov, & Howard, 1977), adolescents with cancer were found to have a less-positive self-image in terms of their social and sexual self. No differences were noted in perceived social support between ill and healthy adolescents. However, many adolescents with cancer reported that they were rejected by their peers and that teachers had lower expectations of them. The isolation and loss of peer support can be more distressing than the threat of disease (Rait & Holland, 1986).

Children with chronic health conditions who experience disease- and treatment-related physical changes are at increased risk for difficulties in peer relations (Spirito, DeLawyer, & Stark, 1991), putting them in a position of potential social vulnerability as a result of being different. In addition, feeling different about their bodies because of sexual development or delayed sexual development secondary to cancer places adolescents with cancer at risk for an altered self-image. Similar to previous investigations that highlighted the use of adaptive denial by adolescents with cancer, Stern et al. (1993) also reported that adolescents with cancer had a tendency to minimize the long-term impact of their illness.

When asked who was their primary support since the time of illness, most adolescents with cancer (77%) identified their mothers (Neville 1993, 1996). When adolescents did not report their mothers as the primary support, they frequently reported becoming protective of their mothers. The previously described case of the 18-year-old male who stated how upset his mother was and how he tried to make the situation easier for her illustrates this. He reported his primary support as his older sister. In another case, a 22-year-old female who recently had been diagnosed with Hodgkin's disease described her boyfriend and aunt as being most supportive and helpful.

"I don't talk to my parents first. I don't want to get them upset. They can't get this thing under control. Like this morning, they knew I was coming in for chemotherapy, and they kept asking if I was nervous or upset. Sure I was, but I said no. I try to be supportive of them. My boyfriend is always there for me. He stays over because nights are really bad. I wake up from nightmares, and he's there to talk to me. My aunt is great. You see, I haven't been able to work at all for two months, and she gives me money and everything."

Adolescents reported their fathers as the next most helpful and supportive, followed by siblings. In one case, a male who had a younger sister who had been treated for cancer two years earlier reported her to be the most helpful and supportive because she shared her experience with him.

Overall findings revealed that the immediate family provided the majority of support for adolescents recently diagnosed with cancer (Neville, 1993). Aunts and uncles, grandparents, girlfriends or boyfriends, friends, and healthcare professionals were additional sources of support. God, godparents, stepparents, and family friends also were mentioned as supports.

In the study, less than half of the adolescents (45%) reported that their friends reacted in a supportive manner to their illness. Adolescents stated that their friends called frequently, sent or brought gifts to the hospital and home, kept them abreast of school and social activities, participated in fund-raising activities, and verbalized concern for them. One 16-year-old male described his friends' reaction when he told them of his illness. "My friends felt bad that it had to happen to me. They consider me an OK guy. At first they laughed when I told them I had it in my testicle and it had spread to my lung. Then they got serious and believed me. Now they call a lot."

Approximately 25% of the adolescents in this study described their friends as "shocked" about their illness, citing initial disbelief and inability to understand how they developed cancer. Some adolescents described their friends as being "no different" and treating them the same as always. A small number of adolescents reported that their friends became more aware of their own physical health status and made efforts to prevent colds, maintain good nutrition, avoid the sun, and obtain sufficient rest. Only two adolescents reported that their friends avoided them. One adolescent said, "They took it funny. I guess they don't know what to ask, what to say, or how to act, so I guess they just stay away."

Overall, most adolescents reported that their friends and peers were very upset initially and then tried to be helpful. Several related their discontent about being the focus of their families' concern and discussion. One 16-year-old female who had been diagnosed with malignant melanoma described the stigma that is frequently associated with cancer and her small town's reaction to her illness. "My whole town is talking about me. They say things like they saw me at the beach getting tan. The illnesses that I have range from a brain tumor to the flu. My real friends know how I am, but there are so many rumors."

The Influence of Culture and Gender on Social Support

In a comparative study between African American and Caucasian families of children with chronic illnesses, Williams (1993) found differences in types of support received. Caucasian families identified affective support as their primary support. African American families identified instrumental types of support.

Neville (1993, 1996) compared differences in perceived social support between male and female adolescents with cancer. Statistically significant differences were noted, with females reporting higher levels of perceived social support. Even among younger children with cancer, girls perceived higher parental social support and higher social support from friends (Varni, Katz, Colegrove, & Dolgin, 1994). These findings are consistent with previous reports (Burke & Weir, 1978) that healthy adolescent females were more likely to inform friends of their problems, felt more comfortable discussing their problems with peers, and were more satisfied with their peers as helpers. Society's general acceptance of females sharing, revealing, and discussing emotional and personal issues may have influenced these findings .

These findings, which are consistent with the work of Chodorow (1974) and Gilligan (1982), may relate to feministic theory. Chodorow describes a sex difference in relationships that occurs during the early years of childhood. As a result of parenting from the same sex during individuation, women come to see themselves as very connected to the world, with a high degree of empathy for the needs and feelings of others. Gilligan also supports the idea that women experience relationships differently than men. During the development of gender identity, masculinity requires separation from the mother. Females, however, develop femininity through attachment to a person of the same sex. Males, according to Gilligan, tend to have problems with relationships, and females tend to have problems with individuation. In the life cycle, identity and intimacy are intertwined. Women learn to know and define themselves through their relationships with and concern for others. The increased perception of social support reported by adolescent females in these studies supports Gilligan's proposition that a greater sense of affiliation and connectedness with others exists through relationships.

The Effect of Social Support on Psychosocial Adjustment

Social support functions to reduce uncertainty during life crises by providing feedback about the meaning of events (Wortman & Dunkel-Schetter, 1979). Having opportunities to discuss and clarify contingencies with others through supportive interactions assists people in forming a cognitive schema (Wortman, 1984). Through these interactions, an individual can gain information regarding the perception of a threatening situation and/or about the resources to cope with the situation.

Although social support has been recognized as an important component in helping to buffer the effects of stressful life events during health and illness states, less research has focused specifically on how increased social support improves health and well-being. Substantial research has documented the positive effect of social support on facilitating the psychosocial adjustment of patients with cancer and their families. Investigators have suggested the need to examine the influence of intervening and mediating or third factors on social support and psychological distress (Bloom, 1990; Holahan & Moos, 1981). Further investigation of these third factors may shed important light on associating factors related to these two variables.

Neville (1993, 1998) examined the relationships between uncertainty, social support, and psychological distress among adolescents recently diagnosed with cancer. When the relationships between perceived social support and psychological distress were examined, a statistically significant, albeit weak, inverse relationship was noted. This finding is consistent with adult cancer research that found that having others with whom to interact and share opinions during illness has a positive impact on psychological distress (Mishel & Braden, 1987). People perceive one form of social support as being cared for in the family and work environment. This perception has been related to lower levels of depression (Holahan & Moos, 1981).

Perceived social support and psychological adjustment also have been studied in families of children with cancer. During the treatment phase, positive correlations existed between various sources of support and parents' psychological adjustment; but, after treatment, only support provided by relatives was found to aid parental adjustment (Morrow, Carpenter, & Hoagland, 1984). This finding is consistent with outcomes of many studies that view social support as a process and attest to its changing nature. In addition, Kupst and Schulman (1988) found that parents who were "good copers" tended to have better support from family members.

Research also has found parental differences in perceived social support and psychosocial adjustment in childhood cancer. Speechley and Noh (1992) found that social support is inversely related to parental anxiety and depression for both parents, but perceived social support is of greater importance to women.

Neville (1993, 1998) found a strong relationship between social support and uncertainty when studying adolescents with cancer. Mishel (1988b) theorized that social support directly modifies uncertainty by reducing ambiguity concerning the state of the illness, the complexity perceived in treatment, and the unpredictability of the future.

In their study of women with gynecologic cancer, Mishel and Braden (1987) identified how these women valued having concerned others listen to them as they expressed their thoughts and feelings. These women stated that having the opportunity to share their perceptions assisted them in obtaining a clearer understanding of their illness. Having others who are willing to discuss the treatment plan reduces anxiety and helps individuals to weigh the options more logically. Mishel and Braden's (1987) theoretical proposition about the indirect effect of social support on uncertainty involves clarification through others regarding the interpretation of symptom patterns. Having others who share information in a social network aids in the appraisal of symptoms during illness (Mishel, 1988b). During research, Neville (1993, 1998) frequently witnessed sharing of information regarding symptoms among adolescents and their parents. Long hours were spent in the pediatric day hospital while participants underwent chemotherapy treatments, waited for examinations, and discussed test results. Here, social networks were formed among families. These small groups were able to provide additional information about symptoms, diagnostic workups, treatments, and responses to therapy. Adolescents shared similarities with each other as they exchanged stories regarding the physical aspects of treatment, their illnesses, and hospital experiences. Overall, families most often provided social support functions to reduce uncertainty in illness, which is consistent with previous studies.

Methodology and Data Analysis in Social Support Research

Numerous researchers have documented the appraisal of uncertainty as a negative event with resultant anxiety (Wong & Bramwell, 1992), psychological distress (Campbell, 1986; Mishel & Braden, 1987; Mishel, Hostetter, King, & Graham, 1984), and coping (Sterken, 1996). Neville (1993, 1998) also found a strong relationship between uncertainty and psychological distress. The research methodology that Neville used will be discussed to illustrate the complex nature of quantitative research. With 60 adolescents, each of the variables in this study: uncertainty, social support, and psychological distress—initially were investigated and scored. After the bivariate relationships of uncertainty, social support, and psychological distress had been established, multiple regression analyses using SPSS® statistical software were conducted to determine the predictive variance of each independent variable on psychological distress (Neville, 1993, 1998). In essence, the influence of uncertainty and social support on predicting psychological distress was being sought. Uncertainty was found to be a significant predictor of psychological distress, but social support was not.

An interaction effect between uncertainty and perceived social support on psychological distress then was investigated. After the initial analyses, comparative analysis was done to compare adolescents with varying levels of social support and uncertainty. A significant interaction effect between uncertainty and social support was found to be the most significant predictor of psychological distress and, combined, accounted for 39% of the variance in psychological distress. To help to interpret this data, the uncertainty and social support scores were dichotomized into high and low scores at the median point and resulting cell means of psychological distress (see Table 2-1). In this study, a high level of uncertainty in illness combined with a low level of social support significantly explained the greatest variance in psychological distress. Adolescents who had the greatest amount of uncertainty and low levels of social support manifested the greatest amount of psychological distress. This finding supports the belief that positive outcomes are implicit in social support.

Table 2-1. Cell Means of Psychological Distress

		Uncertainty	
		Low	High
Perceived social support	Low	n = 13 M = 0.51	n = 19 M = 0.96
	High	n = 16 M = 0.58	n = 12 M = 0.89

Although these variables were examined from a cross-sectional perspective and, therefore, somewhat static in measurement, recent research has supported that social support and uncertainty are dynamic processes that change throughout the course of illness (e.g., peer social support has a tendency to lessen throughout time). This has been well-documented in the adolescent cancer literature. The complexities of these psychosocial variables are multiple and intricate, and additional research using theoretical bases is vital to the advancement of knowledge regarding the psychosocial responses to illness.

References

Aro, H., Hanninen, V., & Paronen, O. (1989). Social support, life events, and psychosomatic symptoms among 14–16-year-old adolescents. *Social Science and Medicine, 29,* 1051–1056.

Baider, L., & Kaplan De-Nour, A. (1989). Group therapy with adolescent cancer patients. *Journal of Adolescent Healthcare, 10,* 35–38.

Baum, B., & Baum, E. (1990). Psychosocial challenges of childhood cancer. *Journal of Psychosocial Oncology, 7,* 119–129.

Bearison, D., & Pacifici, C. (1984). Psychological studies of children who have cancer. *Journal of Applied Developmental Psychology, 5,* 263–280.

Belenky, M., Clinchy, B., Goldberger, N., & Tarule, J. (1986). *Women's way of knowing: The development of self, voice, and mind.* New York: Basic Books.

Binger, C., Ablin, A., Feuerstein, R., Kushner, J., Zoger, S., & Mikkelsen, C. (1969). Childhood leukemia: Emotional impact on the child and family. *New England Journal of Medicine, 280,* 414–419.

Blackmore, C. (1988). The impact of orchidectomy upon the sexuality of the man with testicular cancer. *Cancer Nursing, 11,* 33–40.

Bloom, J. (1990). The relationship of social support and health. *Social Science and Medicine, 30,* 635–637.

Blotcky, A., & Cohen, D. (1985). Psychological assessment of the adolescent with cancer. *Journal of the Association of Pediatric Oncology Nurses, 2,* 8–14.

Bluebond-Langner, M. (1978). *The private worlds of dying children.* Princeton, NJ: Princeton University Press.

Bruhn, J., & Philips, B. (1984). Measuring social support. A synthesis of current approaches. *Journal of Behavioral Medicine, 7,* 151–169.

Brunnquell, D., & Hall, M. (1982). Issues in the psychological care of pediatric oncology patients. *American Journal of Orthopsychiatry, 50,* 32–44.

Budner, S. (1962). Intolerance of ambiguity as a personality variable. *Journal of Personality, 20,* 29–50.

Burke, R., & Weir, T. (1978). Sex differences in adolescent life stress, social support, and well-being. *Journal of Psychology, 98,* 277–288.

Campbell, L. (1986). *Hopelessness and uncertainty as predictors of psychosocial adjustment of newly diagnosed cancer patients and their significant others.* Unpublished doctoral dissertation, The University of Texas at Austin.

Caplan, G. (1974). Support systems. In G. Caplan (Ed.), *Support systems and community mental health: Lectures on concept development* (pp. 1–8). New York: Behavioral Publications.

Carr-Gregg, M., & White, L. (1987). The adolescent with cancer: A psychological overview. *Medical Journal of Australia, 10,* 496–502.

Chodorow, N. (1974). Family structure and feminine personality. In M.Z. Rosaldo & L. Lamphere (Eds.), *Woman, culture, and society* (pp. 43–66). Stanford, CA: Stanford University Press.

Christman, N., McConnell, E., Pfeiffer, C., Webster, K., Schmidt, M., & Rics, J. (1988). Uncertainty, coping, and distress following myocardial infarction: Transition from hospital to home. *Research in Nursing and Health, 11*(2), 71–82.

Clarke-Steffen, L. (1993). Waiting and not knowing: The diagnosis of cancer in a child. *Journal of Pediatric Oncology Nursing, 10,* 146–153.

Cobb, S. (1976). Social support as a moderator of life stress. *Psychosomatic Medicine, 38,* 300–314.

Cohen, D., & Klopovich, P. (1986). The adolescent with cancer. Introduction. *Seminars in Oncology Nursing, 2,* 73–74.

Cohen, M. (1993). The unknown and the unknowable—Managing sustained uncertainty. *Western Journal of Nursing Research, 15,* 77–96.

Cohen, M., & Martinson, I. (1988). Chronic uncertainty: Its effects on parental appraisal of a child's health. *Journal of Pediatric Nursing, 3,* 89–96.

Comaroff, M., & Maguire, P. (1981). Ambiguity and the search for meaning: Childhood leukemia in the modern clinical context. *Social Science and Medicine, 15B,* 115–123.

Craig, T., & Abeloff, M. (1974). Psychiatric symptomatology among hospitalized cancer patients. *American Journal of Psychiatry, 141,* 1323–1327.

Derogatis, L. (1977). *SCL-90-R: Administration, scoring, and procedure manual I.* Baltimore: Clinical Psychometric Research.

Derogatis, L. (1986). The psychosocial adjustment of illness scale. *Journal of Psychosomatic Research, 30,* 77–91.

Derogatis, L., & Melisaratos, N. (1983). The Brief Symptom Inventory: An introductory report. *Psychological Medicine, 13,* 595–605.

Derogatis, L., Morrow, G., Fetting, J., Penman, D., Piasetsky, S., Schmale, A., Henrichs, M., & Carnicke, C. (1983). The prevalence of psychiatric disorders among cancer patients. *JAMA, 249,* 751–757.

Derogatis, L., & Spencer, P. (1982). *Administration and procedures: BSI manual I.* Baltimore: Clinical Psychometric Research.

Elkind, D. (1985). Cognitive development and adolescent disabilities. *Journal of Adolescent Health Care, 6,* 84–89.

Ganz, P. (1988). Patient education as a moderator of psychological distress. *Journal of Psychosocial Oncology, 6,* 181–197.

Gilligan, C. (1982). *In a different voice.* Cambridge, MA: Harvard University Press.

Hinds, P. (1997). Revising theories on adolescent development through observations by nurses. *Journal of Pediatric Oncology Nursing, 14,* 1–2.

Holahan, C., & Moos, R. (1981). Social support and psychological distress. *Journal of Abnormal Psychology, 90,* 365–370.

Kellerman, J., Zeltzer, L., Ellenberg, L., Dash, J., & Rigler, D. (1980). Psychological effects of illness in adolescence. I. Anxiety, self-esteem, and perception of control. *Journal of Pediatrics, 97,* 126–131.

Koocher, G. (1985). Psychosocial care of the child cured of cancer. *Pediatric Nursing, 11*(2), 91–93.

Koocher, G., & O'Malley, J. (1981). *The Damocles syndrome: Psychological consequences of surviving childhood cancer.* New York: McGraw-Hill.

Krishnasamy, M. (1996). Social support and the patient with cancer: A consideration of the literature. *Journal of Advanced Nursing, 23*, 757–762.

Kupst, M. (1994). Coping with pediatric cancer: Theoretical and research perspectives. In D.J. Bearison & R.K. Mulhern (Eds.), *Pediatric psychooncology: Psychological perspectives on children with cancer.* New York: Oxford University Press.

Kupst, M., & Schulman, J. (1988). Long-term coping with pediatric leukemia: A six-year follow-up study. *Journal of Pediatric Psychology, 13*, 7–22.

Levenson, P., Pfefferbaum, B., Copeland, D., & Silberberg, Y. (1982). Information preferences of cancer patients ages 11–20 years. *Journal of Adolescent Health Care, 3*, 9–13.

Lowenberg, J. (1970). The coping behavior of fatally ill adolescents and their parents. *Nursing Forum, 9*, 269–287.

Martinson, I. (1976). *Home care of the dying child: Professional and family perspectives.* Norwalk, CT: Appleton-Century-Crofts.

Martinson, I., & Cohen, M. (1988). Themes from a longitudinal study of family reaction to childhood cancer. *Journal of Psychosocial Oncology, 6*, 81–98.

Mishel, M. (1981a). The measurement of uncertainty in illness. *Nursing Research, 30*, 258–263.

Mishel, M. (1981b). *Perceived ambiguity of events associated with the experience of illness and hospitalization: Development and testing of a measurement tool.* Unpublished doctoral dissertation, Claremont Graduate College, Claremont, CA.

Mishel, M. (1988a). Coping with uncertainty in illness situation. Proceedings of conference: *Stress, coping processes, and health outcomes: New directions in theory development and research* (pp. 51–84). Rochester, NY: Sigma Theta Tau International, Epsilon XI Chapter, University of Rochester.

Mishel, M. (1988b). Uncertainty in illness. *Image: Journal of Nursing Scholarship, 20*, 225–232.

Mishel, M. (1990). Reconceptualization of the uncertainty in illness theory. *Image: Journal of Nursing Scholarship, 22*, 256–262.

Mishel, M., & Braden, C. (1987). Uncertainty: A mediator between support and adjustment. *Western Journal of Nursing Research, 9*, 43–57.

Mishel, M., & Braden, C. (1988). Finding meaning: Antecedents of uncertainty in illness. *Nursing Research, 37*, 98–107, 127.

Mishel, M., & Epstein, D. (1990). *Uncertainty in Illness Scale manual.* Unpublished manuscript.

Mishel, M., Hostetter, T., King, B., & Graham, V. (1984). Predictors of psychological adjustment in patients newly diagnosed with cancer. *Cancer Nursing, 1*, 291–299.

Moore, D., Holton, C., & Martin, G. (1969). Psychological problems in the management of adolescents with malignancy. *Clinical Pediatrics, 8*, 464–473.

Morrow, G., Carpenter, P., & Hoagland, A. (1984). The role of social support in parental adjustment to pediatric cancer. *Journal of Pediatric Psychology, 9*, 317–329.

Neville, K. (1993). *The relationships among perceived social support, uncertainty, and psychological distress of male and female adolescents recently diagnosed with cancer.* Unpublished doctoral dissertation, New York University.

Neville, K. (1996). Psychological distress in adolescents with cancer. *Journal of Pediatric Nursing, 11*, 243–251.

Neville, K. (1998). The relationships among uncertainty, perceived social support, and psychosocial distress in adolescents recently diagnosed with cancer. *Journal of Pediatric Oncology Nursing, 15*, 37–46.

Nightingale, F. (1992). *Notes on nursing: What it is, and what it is not* [Commemorative edition]. Philadelphia: J.B. Lippincott.

Offer, D., Ostrov, E., & Howard, K. (1977). *A manual for the Offer Self-Image Questionnaire for adolescents.* Chicago: Michael Reese Hospital and Medical Center.

Ostrov, E., Offer, D., & Howard, K. (1989). Gender differences in adolescent symptomatology: A normative study. *Journal of the Academy of Child and Adolescent Psychiatry, 28,* 394–398.

Parsons, T. (1980). Health, uncertainty, and the action situation. In S. Fiddle (Ed.), *Uncertainty: Behavioral and social dimensions* (pp. 145–162). New York: Praeger.

Rait, P., & Holland, J. (1986). Pediatric cancer: Psychosocial issues and approaches. *Mediguide to Oncology, 6,* 1–6.

Rosenberg, M. (1965). *Society and the adolescent self-image.* Princeton, NJ: Princeton University Press.

Speechley, K., & Noh, S. (1992). Surviving childhood cancer, social support, and parents' psychological adjustment. *Journal of Pediatric Psychology, 17,* 15–31.

Speilberger, C., Gorsuch, R., & Lushene, R. (1970). *STAI manual for the State-Trait Anxiety Inventory.* Palo Alto, CA: Consulting Psychologists.

Spirito, A., DeLawyer, D., & Stark, L. (1991). Peer relations and social adjustment of chronically ill children and adolescents. *Clinical Psychology Review, 11,* 539–564.

Sterken, D. (1996). Uncertainty and coping in fathers of children with cancer. *Journal of Pediatric Oncology Nursing, 13,* 81–88.

Stern, M., Norman, S., & Zevon, M. (1993). Adolescents with cancer: Self-image and perceived social support as indexes of adaptation. *Journal of Adolescent Research, 8,* 124–142.

Stovall, A., & Peacock, M. (1984). The family of the adolescent with cancer. *Cancer Bulletin, 36,* 285–288.

Tebbi, C., Stern, M., Boyle, M., Mettlin, C., & Mindell, E. (1985). The role of social support systems in adolescent amputee cancer patients. *Cancer, 56,* 965–971.

Van Dongen-Melman, J., Pruyn, J., Van Zanen, G., & Sanders-Woudstra, J. (1986). Coping with childhood cancer: A conceptual view. *Journal of Psychosocial Oncology, 4,* 147–161.

Varni, J., Katz, E., Colegrove, R., & Dolgin, M. (1994). Perceived social support and adjustment of children with newly diagnosed cancer. *Developmental and Behavioral Pediatrics, 15,* 20–26.

Vessey, J., & Swanson, M. (1996). Chronic conditions and child development. In P. Jackson & J. Vessey (Eds.), *Primary care of the child with a chronic condition* (2nd ed.) (pp. 16–39). St. Louis: Mosby.

Wallston, B., Wallston, K., Kaplan, G., & Maides, S. (1976). Development and validation of the Health and Locus of Control Scale. *Journal of Consulting and Clinical Psychology, 44,* 580.

Weekes, D. (1989). *Adolescents with cancer: Correlates of intraindividual change in types of coping strategy.* Unpublished doctoral dissertation, University of California, San Francisco.

Weisman, A., & Worden, J. (1976–77). The existential plight in cancer: Significance of the first 100 days. *International Journal of Psychiatry in Medicine, 7,* 1–15.

Weiss, R. (1974). The provision of social relationships. In R. Zick (Ed.), *Doing unto others* (pp. 17–26). Englewood Cliffs, NJ: Prentice-Hall.

Williams, H. (1993). A comparison of social support and social network of black parents and white parents with chronically ill children. *Social Science and Medicine, 37,* 1509–1520.

Wong, C., & Bramwell, K. (1992). Uncertainty and anxiety after mastectomy for breast cancer. *Cancer Nursing, 15,* 363–371.

Wool, M., & Goldberg, R. (1986). Assessment of denial in cancer patients: Implications for intervention. *Journal of Psychosocial Oncology, 4,* 1–14.

Wortman, C. (1984). Social support and the cancer patient: Conceptual and methodologic issues. *Cancer, 53*(Suppl. 10), 2339–2362.

Wortman, C., & Dunkel-Schetter, C. (1979). Interpersonal relationships and cancer: A theoretical analysis. *Journal of Social Issues, 35,* 120–155.

Zeltzer, L., Kellerman, J., Ellenberg, L., Dash, J., & Rigler, D. (1980). Psychological effects of illness in adolescence. II. Impact of illness on adolescents—Crucial issues and coping styles. *Journal of Pediatrics, 97,* 132–138.

Zeltzer, L., LeBaron, S., & Zeltzer, P. (1984). The adolescent with cancer. In R.W. Blum (Ed.), *Chronic illness and disabilities in childhood and adolescence* (pp. 375–395). New York: Grune & Stratton.

Zevon, M., Tebbi, C., & Stern, M. (1987). Psychological and familial factors in adolescent oncology. In C. Tebbi (Ed.), *Major topics in adolescent oncology* (pp. 325–349). Mount Kisco, NY: Futura.

CHAPTER 3.
Overview of Cancer in Children and Adolescents

Mary McElwain Petriccione, RN, MSN, PNP

Introduction

Pediatric cancers are a unique group of malignancies that differ significantly from adult cancers. Their clinical, biologic, and genetic components have contributed greatly to an increased understanding of malignant transformation, particularly in the area of genetics (Marina, 1997).

The emergence of pediatric oncology as a distinct specialty has led to increased treatment success. In 1934 in New York City, Memorial Hospital opened the first children's cancer ward, a four-bed unit. In 1950, the unit expanded to 26 beds. In the 1960s, St. Jude Children's Research Hospital opened in Memphis, TN. It was the first hospital to treat childhood malignancies exclusively (Foley & Fergusson, 1993). The care of children with cancer became increasingly multidisciplinary. New treatments evolved with the advent of the multiple modality approach to a disease entity. Nationwide cooperative study groups emerged in an attempt to formalize and analyze the treatment approaches to specific diseases. The Children's Cancer Group (CCG) and the Pediatric Oncology Group (POG), the two main research groups, have now combined their efforts and are called the Children's Oncology Group (COG). In 1974, the Association of Pediatric Oncology Nurses (APON) was founded. Both the medical and nursing professions were recognizing pediatric oncology as a specialty. Improved standardized quality of care for children and adolescents was the result.

Overview

Cancer is the second leading cause of death among children 1–14 years of age in the United States, with accidents being the first (Landis, Murray, Bolden, & Wingo, 1999). More children die from cancer, however, than any other disease. Approximately 11,000 children and teenagers are diagnosed with cancer each year, with an increasing incidence rate of approximately 1% each year. The most common cancers found in children are leukemias (particularly acute lymphocytic leukemia), brain and other nervous system cancers, non-Hodgkin's lymphoma (NHL), and soft tissue cancers (Landis et al.). Significant improvements have been made in 5-year relative survival rates throughout the past 20 years (see Table 3-1). Between 1974 and 1994, survival rates improved by at least 20% for leukemia (acute lymphocytic and myeloid), central nervous system tumors, NHL, and Wilms' tumor (see Table 3-1) (Landis et al.).

Table 3-1. Trends in Cancer Survival for Children Under 15 Years of Age in United States From 1974–1994

Sites	Five-Year Relative Survival Rates (%)					
	Year of Diagnosis					
	1974–1976	1977–1979	1980–1982	1983–1985	1986–1988	1989–1994
All sites	56	62	65	68	70	74 [a]
Acute lymphocytic leukemia	53	67	70	70	78	80 [a]
Acute myeloid leukemia	14	20 [b]	21 [b]	32 [b]	28 [b]	43 [a]
Bones and joints	54 [b]	53 [b]	54 [b]	59 [b]	62 [b]	64 [a]
Brain and other nervous system disorders	55	56	55	62	62	83 [a]
Hodgkin's disease	79	83	91	90	90	92 [a]
Neuroblastoma	52	54	53	54	60	69 [a]
Non-Hodgkin's lymphoma	45	51	62	70	69	78 [a]
Soft tissue	61	69	65	78	66	76 [a]
Wilms' tumor	74	77	87	86	91	92 [a]

[a] The difference in rates between 1974–1976 and 1989–1994 is statistically significant ($p < 0.05$).
[b] The standard error of the survival rate is between 5 and 10 percentage points.

Note. All sites exclude basal and squamous cell skin cancers and *in situ* carcinomas except urinary bladder. Based on information from the National Cancer Institute Surveillance, Epidemiology, and End Results Program, 1996.

Note. From "Cancer Statistics, 1999," by S.H. Landis, T. Murray, S. Bolden, and P.A. Wingo, 1999, *CA: A Cancer Journal for Clinicians, 49*, p. 31. Copyright 1999 by Lippincott-Raven Publishers. Reprinted with permission.

Etiologic Factors Associated With Cancer in Children and Adolescents

The exact causes of childhood cancer are not known. A small percentage of specific diseases (e.g., leukemia, Down syndrome, low-grade gliomas and neurofibromatosis) can be associated with chromosomal and genetic abnormalities. Environmental factors are suspect, but direct correlations have been difficult to support. In a small number of cases (e.g., ionizing radiation and brain tumors), strong associations can be made (Wartenburg, 1996). Validating these numbers is difficult because accurately determining children's exposure levels after the cancer has developed is not possible. The overall small number of children diagnosed each year makes a large study impossible. Associations have been made between maternal drug exposure and tumor development (e.g., phenytoin and neuroblastoma). Associations between viruses and cancer (e.g., the Epstein-Barr virus [EBV] and

NHL and Hodgkin's disease) have been found in individuals who are immunosuppressed and, less consistently, those who are not (Razzouk, Srinivas, Sample, Singh, & Sixbey, 1996). Much research is focused on the role that all of these factors play in the development of childhood cancers as well as parental occupational exposures, parental medical conditions before conception or during pregnancy, and parental, fetal, or childhood exposures to environmental and household toxins.

Children infected with HIV are being studied to determine whether their cancer risk is greater than in the noninfected population. These children, in addition to having profound immune system dysfunction, also may be infected with potentially oncogenic viruses (e.g., EBV, human papilloma virus, hepatitis B virus) (Mueller & Pizzo, 1997). The most common neoplasms diagnosed in these children include lymphoma, Kaposi's sarcoma, and leiomyosarcoma.

A "cluster" of cancers occasionally are diagnosed in a particular area. The investigation by the state and local health department usually determines that the number of new cases does not exceed the pattern in the overall population. Cases have been documented, however, in which environmental or chemical toxicities are concentrated in a small area, with strong correlations made between population exposure and cancer development. Incidences such as these illustrate the need for more epidemiologic research on a larger systematic scale so that harmful toxins can be identified and handled appropriately.

Treatment Interventions for Children and Adolescents With Cancer

All children diagnosed with cancer should be treated in a pediatric cancer center. Studies have shown that children treated in such centers have increased event-free survival (Sanders et al., 1997). Specialized centers have standardized treatment protocols that ensure that children expeditiously receive a comprehensive workup and evaluation of all pertinent data by a multidisciplinary oncology team. Once an accurate diagnosis is made, including pertinent staging, children are entered in a clinical trial, when possible, so that state-of-the-art treatment can be given, monitored, and analyzed. Follow-up after the completion of therapy includes monitoring for disease recurrence and long-term effects. In this way, each child is guaranteed to receive the best possible care and is contributing information to the treatment of specific diseases.

Advances in many facets of treatment have dramatically improved the care of children with cancer and had a positive impact on the length and quality of survival. New imaging techniques have improved the diagnostic process with increased speed, accuracy, and information. For example, the use of magnetic resonance imaging (MRI) provides detailed physiologic and anatomic data, including evaluation of vascular structures, without using IV contrast (Prados, Berger, & Wilson, 1998). Although paramagnetic contrast (gadolinium-DTPA) is used when evaluating central nervous system tumors, the role of contrast in extracranial tumors continues to be investigated (Parker, 1997). Studies such as the positron emission tomography (PET) and magnetic resonance spectroscopy (MRS) are giving more information when a tumor recurrence is in question. Functional MRI is capable of pinpointing critical areas of brain function. Sophisticated imaging studies are a necessity throughout all stages of treatment, particularly if disease recurrence becomes an issue.

Surgical intervention is a vital treatment modality of many protocols. The specific surgical intervention that is required depends on the disease, and its complexity can range from a biopsy to a resection of varying degrees. Advances in technique and intraoperative monitoring now have made possible complete tumor resections in vital areas while maintaining all or most of normal functioning (Prados et al., 1998). The goal of using the least invasive surgical procedure along with improved reconstructive surgical techniques has resulted in increased function for many patients. Surgically implanting venous access devices (e.g., infusaport) has allowed the safe infusion of a wide variety of agents to patients with fragile veins. The role of surgery is invaluable in the "second look" treatment phase to evaluate and remove remaining disease. In certain cases of metastatic or recurrent disease, surgical procedures can improve the chances of a second remission or provide palliative symptomatic relief (Holcomb et al., 1995).

Irradiation is used to achieve high rates of disease control (Lombardi, Navarria, & Gandola, 1998) and is included in various phases of a treatment protocol. A variety of factors, including the disease, its stage, and children's age, determine the dosage and manner of administration. Treatment is administered once or twice a day (hyperfractitionated), five days in succession, for a range of two to six weeks, depending on the total required dose. The most common method of administering irradiation is through external beam. Children must cooperate completely so that the radiation target area is precisely treated. With very young or anxious children, sedation may be necessary to ensure that they remain very still during the treatment, which allows safe and accurate delivery. Radiation therapy also can be delivered intraoperatively in a single dose directly to the tumor site. Interstitial radiation therapy, also known as brachytherapy, has been used in pediatrics to treat retinoblastoma and, most recently, soft tissue sarcomas. It involves computerized tomography (CT) guided implantation of radioactive material directly into the tumor bed. Localized irradiation is administered continuously for a few days. The implants then are removed. Irradiation boosts can be administered to tumor areas in this manner without damaging surrounding healthy tissue (Prados et al., 1998). The primary goal of irradiation is to achieve a "cure," but it also can be used to achieve palliation by shrinking recurrent or metastatic disease.

Chemotherapy is used to treat most types of pediatric cancer and can be administered in multiple ways, in varying doses, and at different points in the treatment protocol (Bergeron, 1998). These agents can be administered alone or in combination with other drugs or treatment modalities. Chemotherapy may be administered preoperatively to reduce tumor burden (neoadjuvant chemotherapy) or after the initial surgery or radiation therapy (adjuvant chemotherapy) (Prados & Russo, 1998). It also can be administered directly into an area such as cerebrospinal fluid to eradicate malignant cells (sanctuary therapy). Most treatment protocols begin with an extremely intensive induction phase to rapidly eliminate the majority of the malignant cells. The consolidation phase is next, with intensive therapy to eradicate any remaining disease. Maintenance therapy follows, and children are treated for a predetermined time period to ensure complete eradication of the disease. Each disease entity has specific protocols that govern the administration of therapy. The treatment of some of the most common pediatric cancers will be discussed in more detail later in this chapter.

Chemotherapeutic agents can be classified by chemical structure into six major categories: alkylating agents, antimetabolites, antitumor antibiotics, plant alkaloids, corticosteroids, and miscellaneous agents (e.g., L-asparaginase). Each agent has a specific therapeutic action and is used alone or in combination with other drugs to achieve the most effective disease control. Each drug or combination of drugs has acute and long-term side effects that need to be addressed in detail with the primary caregiver. Children or adolescents should be given age-appropriate information. Many delivery methods, including IV via peripheral access devices, allow direct access to the cerebrospinal fluid. An implantable pump can be used for intraperitoneal, intracavitary, or intraarterial infusions. Ambulatory infusion pumps allow chemotherapy and hydration to infuse at a set rate throughout a longer time period. Chemotherapy also can be administered orally, intrathecally (directed into the spinal fluid via a lumbar puncture), subcutaneously, or via intramuscular injection.

Researchers have focused on determining the highest, most effective doses of chemotherapeutic agents that can be tolerated while developing methods to circumvent drug-induced toxicity (Balis, Hokenberg, & Poplack, 1997). Historically, protocols including myeloablative doses of chemotherapy, with or without irradiation, have been used for autologous or allogeneic bone marrow transplantation. The reinfusion of autologous peripheral stem cells after myeloablative chemotherapy has become increasingly successful during approximately the past seven years and now is implemented in the outpatient setting. This allows for very high doses of a chemotherapeutic agent (e.g., thiotepa) or combination of agents, such as the high-dose P-C-V protocol (procarbazine, CCNU [lomustine], and vincristine) to be administered. Patients then receive a reinfusion of autologous peripheral blood stem cells, which lessens the period of pancytopenia (Dunkel et al., 1998). Granulocyte-colony-stimulating factor (G-CSF) is administered to further promote the recovery of the white blood cell count. As with all chemotherapeutic protocols, intensive supportive care is imperative with this regimen. The administration of antiemetics, irradiated blood products, hydration fluid, pain medication, antibiotics, and antiviral and antifungal agents as needed will lessen anticipated toxicities and complications from therapy. The role of nurses in providing comprehensive patient and family education is paramount so that patients have the knowledge they need to confront and cope with treatment-related effects.

Leukemia

Overview

Leukemia represents approximately 39% of childhood and adolescent cancers, making it the most common malignancy in this age group (Magrath et al., 1996). Approximately 3,000 new cases are diagnosed each year, with approximately 80% of the cases diagnosed as acute lymphocytic leukemia (ALL) and 20% of the cases as acute myeloid leukemia (AML) (Robinson, 1997). Chronic myelogenous leukemia is rare. Childhood leukemia is more common in boys than girls and in whites than blacks (Margolin & Poplack, 1997). The treatment of leukemia has improved so dramatically that survival rates have gone from approximately 4% in the 1960s to an overall cure rate of 75% in 1999. The cure rate is now as high as 95% in children with certain positive cytogenetic characteristics in their leukemia.

Etiologic Factors Associated With Leukemia in Children

Researchers have spent much time trying to determine the cause of leukemia. ALL is linked to a strong genetic component. Constitutional chromosomal abnormalities and fragility syndromes associated with increased risk of childhood leukemia include trisomy 21, Bloom syndrome, Fanconi's anemia, ataxia-telangiectasia, neurofibromatosis, Schwachman syndrome, and, rarely, Klinefelter's syndrome (Friebert & Shurin, 1998; Shannon, 1998). Exposure to environmental agents (e.g., radiation, chemicals, drugs, pesticides) also may lead to leukemia. The only clear associations that have been made are with exposures to therapeutic and other forms of ionizing radiation and certain toxic chemicals (e.g., benzene, some chemotherapeutic agents) (Friebert & Shurin). Ionizing radiation in high doses can cause cell death by inhibiting normal cell division. The degree of exposure to all forms of this type of radiation (e.g., x-rays, radioisotopes) should be limited to certain safe amounts as recommended by the National Council on Radiation Protection and Measurements. Infectious causes of leukemia (e.g., exposures to viruses) have not been proven but are suspect. Siblings of children with leukemia are two to four times more likely to develop the disease than children among the average population. An identical twin has a 25% chance of developing the disease in the first year, with a proportionate decrease in risk with increasing age up to age seven (Friebert & Shurin).

Leukemia does not have standardized staging, but patients are treated according to "risk" groups, which clearly are defined by clinical and laboratory features that are present at diagnosis. These multiple variables include age; white blood cell count; sex; race; presence of central nervous system disease, hepatomegaly, splenomegaly, mediastinal mass, and lymphadenopathy; platelet count; hemoglobin; immunoglobulin levels; rapidity of treatment response; morphology of the blast cells (from the French-American-British [FAB] criteria); immunophenotype; chromosome DNA content (ploidy); specific chromosomal translocations; and nutritional status (Margolin & Poplack, 1997; Pui & Crist, 1994; Steinherz et al., 1996). The presence of these variables differs in each case.

The lymphocyte cell line is involved in ALL. The cellular classification of leukemic cells has a significant impact on treatment and prognosis. This system is based on the cellular characteristics relating to the thymic (T cell) and bursal equivalent (B cell) origin of normal lymphocytes (Gaddy-Cohen, 1993). These leukemic cells are classified according to morphology, immunologic characteristics, and cytogenetics. Thus, identifying the major subgroups of ALL (T cell, B cell, early pre-B cell, and pre-B cell) is possible (Margolin & Poplack).

The morphology of the leukemic cells, which includes form, structure, and cytochemistry, is the basis for one classification criterion. The FABCG criterion identifies the following morphology: L1 morphology present in 80%–85% of patients, L2 morphology present in 15% of cases, and L3 morphology present in 1%–3% of cases. The different cell types are designated on the basis of light microscopic features including size of the cell and nuclear-to-cytoplasm ratio (Friebert & Shurin, 1998). In general, L1 morphology, the type of cell most commonly found in childhood ALL, yields a better prognosis than the L2 morphology. L3 morphology is associated with B cell lineage (Burkitt's-type leukemia) and is treated differently from the other two types (Pui & Crist, 1994; Pui & Evans, 1998).

Immunologic and molecular characterization of the leukemic cell of B and T cell precursors further define the disease. Approximately 80%–85% of childhood ALL cases develop as a result of the proliferation of non-B cell precursors (Margolin & Poplack, 1997). The presence of a common ALL surface antigen (cALLa) is associated with a favorable outcome. The three major subtypes of the B cell precursor to ALL are early pre-B cell, pre-B cell, and B cell. In general, early pre-B cells are present in approximately two-thirds of patients and have the most favorable outcome. They do not have evidence of immunoglobulin and are positive for CALLA (Margolin & Poplack). The pre-B cells are present in approximately 20%–30% of cases of B cell precursors to ALL. These cells possess cytoplasmic immunoglobulin and represent an intermediate cell in the process of B cell differentiation. Their prognosis is not as favorable as the early pre-B set, especially if the chromosomal translocation + (1,19) is present (Margolin & Poplack). Surface immunoglobulin is present in the B cell subset, which represents a mature cell in the differentiation process. It is present in only a very small percentage of children and is indicative of a poor prognosis (Gaddy-Cohen, 1993; Margolin & Poplack).

T cell leukemic cells undergo malignant transformation at various stages along the T lymphocytotic pathway (Gaddy-Cohen, 1993). The presence of CD2, a cell surface antigen, appears to confer a favorable prognosis (Uckun et al., 1996). T cell leukemia is diagnosed predominantly in older children, especially males, and is clinically associated with a high white cell count, mediastinal mass, and hepatosplenomegaly (Uckun, Gaynon, Sensel, et al., 1997). T cell leukemia is an aggressive subtype of ALL and requires intensive treatment.

In as many as 20% of cases, children can present with mixed lineage or biphenotypic leukemia. With this leukemia, the cells have characteristics of both myeloid and lymphoid lineage (Gaddy-Cohen, 1993; Margolin & Poplack, 1997). Two different populations of blast cells with distinct morphology or surface antigens can coexist on the same leukemic cell (Gaddy-Cohen). Whether the prognosis for this type of leukemia treated with current chemotherapeutic protocols is worse than for other similar subsets of ALL is controversial. In a small group of patients with CD2 (a T lineage surface antigen) and CD19 (a B lineage surface antigen), the prognosis was usually good (Uckun, Gaynon, Sather, et al., 1997).

Cytogenetic studies of leukemic cells are performed routinely. Numerical (ploidy) chromosome abnormalities are identified either directly by counting the modal number of chromosomes or indirectly by flow cytometry that measures DNA content (Margolin & Poplack, 1997). Hyperdiploid (>50 chromosomes of DNA index >1.16) is present in approximately 30% of children with ALL and indicates a good prognosis. Structural abnormalities or chromosome substitutions can be determined with molecular techniques such as fluorescence in situ hybridization (FISH) and polymerase chain reaction. The presence of the Philadelphia (Ph) chromosome is a result of translocation + (9, 22) and indicates a poor prognosis (Margolin & Poplack). A chromosome translocation is the shifting of a fragment of one chromosome to another. However, + (12, 21) translocation, which is present in approximately 20% of patients with ALL, indicates a favorable prognosis (Raimondi, 1993).

Clinical Presentation of Leukemia in Children

Children with leukemia can present with a wide range of symptoms and laboratory findings (see Table 3-2). The symptoms usually are present for only a short amount of time, although some patients have reported persistent mild symptoms for as long as several weeks. Children most commonly go to a physician because of bleeding, bruising, or the presence of petechiae, all of which are caused by thrombocytopenia. Fatigue, pallor, increased irritability, and weakness often are experienced and are caused by anemia. Fever of unknown origin or an infection resistant to oral antibiotics (e.g., sinusitis) is another common symptom and is caused by neutropenia. The thrombocytopenia, anemia, and neutropenia are a result of bone marrow failure that occurs when malignant cells invade the bone marrow. Progressive bone or joint pain can result from the rapid expansion of leukemic cells within the marrow space or from bone destruction from leukemic infiltration (Margolin & Poplack, 1997). Anorexia, abdominal pain, weight loss, generalized arthralgias, lymphadenopathy, chronic cough, and simply "looking ill" are other possible symptoms (Friebert & Shurin, 1998; Margolin & Poplack). Patients may have an enlarged liver or spleen as a result of infiltration of leukemic cells. Signs or symptoms of central nervous system involvement are rarely present at the time of diagnosis (Margolin & Poplack). Patients with T cell leukemia, particularly adolescents, can present with persistent cough, facial swelling, and orthopnea, indicating superior vena cava syndrome. This syndrome occurs when a mediastinal mass compresses the superior vena cava or trachea. In children and adolescents, respiratory distress, which worsens if they attempt to lie down, is present. This requires immediate medical attention to improve their ability to aerate effectively (Friebert & Shurin). ALL may mimic a variety of

Table 3-2. Clinical and Laboratory Features at Diagnosis in Children With Acute Lymphocytic Leukemia

Clinical and Laboratory Findings	%
Symptoms and physical findings	
Fever	61
Bleeding (e.g., petechiae, purpura)	48
Bone pain	23
Lymphadenopathy	50
Splenomegaly	63
Hepatosplenomegaly	68
Laboratory features	
Leukocyte count (mm³)	
< 10,000	53
10,000–49,000	30
> 50,000	17
Hemoglobin (g/dl)	
< 7	43
7–11	45
> 11	12
Platelet count (mm³)	
< 20,000	28
20,000–99,000	47
> 100,000	25
Lymphoblast morphology	
L1	84
L2	15
L3	1

Note. From "Acute Lymphoblastic Leukemia" (p. 425) by J.F. Margolin and D.G. Poplack in P.A. Pizzo and D.G. Poplack (Eds.), *Principles and Practice of Pediatric Oncology* (3rd ed.), 1997, Philadelphia: Lippincott-Raven Publishers. Copyright 1997 by Lippincott-Raven Publishers. Reprinted with permission.

nonmalignant conditions (e.g., infectious mononucleosis, aplastic anemia, idiopathic thrombocytopenia purpura) as well as several malignant conditions (e.g., neuroblastoma, lymphoma, rhabdomyosarcoma, retinoblastoma) (Margolin & Poplack).

Diagnostic Workup for Children With Leukemia

Whenever a serious illness is suspected, a thorough physical examination is essential. During the assessment, healthcare professionals should pay particular attention to enlarged nodes, testes, skin, eyes (including a fundoscopic examination), and central nervous system (Friebert & Shurin, 1998; Margolin & Poplack, 1997). The workup should include a complete blood count and examination of the smear. The blood count may be normal, but it usually is not. A white blood cell count greater than 50,000 requires immediate medical attention to prevent leukostasis or metabolic abnormalities (e.g., hyperkalemia, hypocalcemia, hyperuricemia, hyperphosphatemia). Some degree of anemia usually is present with thrombocytopenia. A chemistry panel may reveal a rise in the lactic dehydrogenase (LDH), serum glutamic oxaloacetic tansaminase (SGOT), serum glutamic pyruvic transaminase (SGPT), blood urea nitrogen (BUN), and creatinine. Coagulation studies may or may not be abnormal. An extremely elevated uric acid level (> 10) requires immediate emergency treatment with the use of allopurinol, hydration, and alkalization of the urine. All metabolic abnormalities must be monitored carefully. A chest x-ray is needed to detect the presence of a mediastinal mass, which may need urgent treatment. The lumbar cerebrospinal fluid also must be examined for the presence of leukemic cells. However, evaluation of the bone marrow provides the definitive diagnosis.

A treatment plan then is devised based on prognostic indicators that place patients in a particular risk category (Pui & Crist, 1994; Steinherz et al., 1996). In addition to the cellular prognostic factors discussed earlier in this section, the following features help to determine children's prognoses. Children who are younger than 1 year or older than 10 and those who present with white blood cell counts greater than 50,000, a large tumor burden, or central nervous system disease have a poorer prognosis. T cell leukemia is more aggressive and has a poorer prognosis (Uckun, Gaynon, Sensel, et al., 1997). In general, girls seem to do better than boys, as do children who present with anemia (Gaddy-Cohen, 1993; Margolin & Poplack, 1997). Response to initial "induction" treatment is evolving as an important prognostic indicator. Children or adolescents who quickly clear the marrow or peripheral blood of leukemic blasts (as early as treatment day 7) have an increased chance of long-term event-free survival (Steinherz et al.).

Treatment Interventions for Children With Leukemia

Depending on the specific type of leukemia and the "risk" group to which the disease belongs, treatment strategies differ significantly. Children with ALL are divided into low- and high-risk groups, according to the criteria discussed earlier. This determines the type of chemotherapy administered, the dosage, and the length of treatment time.

Most current treatment protocols are based on several principles: rapid remission induction, consolidation of early intensification (several weeks or months of very aggressive therapy), continued maintenance with combination (multiple drug) chemotherapy, early central nervous system prophylaxis, more intensive initial therapy for "high-risk" groups, and aggressive supportive care (Pui & Crist, 1994). Central nervous system prophylaxis may be achieved with chemotherapy alone, administered intrathecally and systemically in high doses. Cranial low-dose irradiation may be required for "high-risk" patients to prevent central nervous system relapse. Patients who initially present with central nervous system leukemia may require intrathecal chemotherapy to control the disease at diagnosis followed by cranial irradiation.

The aim of induction chemotherapy is to reduce the number of malignant cells in the bone marrow to a level that is not detectable. This allows the normal bone marrow to return and blood counts to return to normal. During this treatment phase, patients who are considered low risk will receive three drugs: prednisone, asparaginase, and vincristine. High-risk patients may receive a fourth drug, usually an anthracycline such as daunorubicin. Central nervous system prophylaxis will be performed with the administration of intrathecal chemotherapy, except for high-risk patients, who will need to undergo cranial irradiation. Most patients achieve a complete remission within the first month of treatment. The presence of > 25% blasts in the bone marrow or persistent blasts in peripheral blood on day 7 of treatment is indicative of a less favorable prognosis (Steinherz et al., 1996). Aggressive supportive care is needed to prevent serious consequences and, in a small percentage of cases, death from infection, hemorrhage, permanent organ damage, tumor lysis syndrome, or metabolic imbalances (Margolin & Poplack, 1997; Nachman et al., 1998).

Once disease is in remission, the consolidation or intensification phase begins and lasts approximately four to eight months. Completely eradicating residual microscopic disease without allowing the remaining cells to become resistant to therapy is important. To achieve this, a combination of several drugs is used. Low- to average-risk patients receive a combination that includes 6-mercaptopurine and intermediate- or high-dose methotrexate (Evans et al., 1998; Harris, Shuster, et al., 1998). Those patients in the high-risk category receive different combinations of drugs at much higher doses (Nachman et al., 1998). The Children's Cancer Group reported their findings from a trial using a modified version of the Berlin-Frankfurt-Munster therapy (which uses an extended intensive consolidation phase) to treat children and adolescents with a poor prognosis. The results showed that an aggressive approach during consolidation can improve the prognosis of poor-risk patients (Nachman et al., 1997).

Maintenance therapy follows consolidation. Most protocols call for daily doses of 6-mercaptopurine, weekly doses of methotrexate, and monthly doses of vincristine and prednisone. Some trials have shown that administering oral 6-mercaptopurine in the evening instead of earlier in the day may improve survival (Schmieglow et al., 1997). Most treatment protocols last for two to three years. Patients must be monitored closely for compliance and evidence of drug toxicity.

Disease relapse can occur during treatment or at any time following completion of treatment. The prognosis depends on many factors, including the time of the relapse. Children or adolescents who relapse while undergoing treatment or shortly thereafter have a more dismal prognosis than those who relapse more than a year from therapy completion. In these cases, aggressive treatment protocols are used. The principal form of treatment failure for patients with ALL is bone marrow relapse (Margolin & Poplack, 1997). Allogeneic marrow transplantation routinely is advocated for patients in second remission who have an appropriate bone marrow donor and have survived a longer, event-free period (Margolin & Poplack). Although the incidence of isolated central nervous system relapse is less common, it still remains a significant cause of treatment failure with a dismal prognosis (Margolin & Poplack; Ribeiro et al., 1995). Males who develop an overt and clinically obvious testicular relapse longer after treatment completion have a better prognosis than those who relapse closer to the end of therapy. Those who develop an occult testicular relapse while off of therapy and are treated aggressively have a similar prognosis to those with an overt relapse.

Future Directions in the Treatment of Children With Leukemia

In the future, researchers will attempt to develop more effective therapy for patients who relapse while following standard protocols and improve methods of disease assessment and treatment so that relapses in the "standard-risk" group can be eradicated. Another priority will be to develop alternative therapies that avoid the dangerous long-term effects caused by radiation (e.g., neurocognitive delays, endocrine dysfunction) and certain genotoxic agents (e.g., VM26), which studies have shown present an increased risk of developing secondary acute myelogenous leukemia (Pui, Evans, & Gilbert, 1998).

Acute Myelogenous Leukemia

Overview

AML represents approximately 15%–20% of all childhood leukemias (Pui et al., 1998). Most incidences of AML occur from 10 years of age through adolescence and at 55 years of age and older. Incidence is distributed equally among ethnic groups. Male-to-female ratio is approximately equal. Minimal geographic differences are noted. Of newly diagnosed children with AML, 75%–85% have their disease go into remission with intensive induction treatment and 40% will be disease free at five years (Hurwitz, Mounce, & Grier, 1995; Pui et al., 1998).

Etiologic Factors Related to Acute Myelogenous Leukemia

The cause of AML is unknown. Although most children diagnosed with AML have no predisposing conditions, some children, including those with various genetic or inherited conditions such as Down syndrome, Fanconi's anemia, Bloom syndrome, Kostmann syndrome, Diamond Blackfan anemia, and neurofibromatosis, are at greater risk for developing the disease (Golub, Weinstein, & Grier, 1997). The identical twin of children with acute leukemia has a 20% risk of developing acute leukemia, particularly before six years of age. Children treated for myelodysplastic syndromes (e.g., aplastic anemia) and those exposed to ionizing radiation or chemicals (e.g., benzene) are at higher risk (Ebb & Weinstein, 1997; Golub et al.). Children treated with alkylating agents, nitrosoureas, and epipodophyllotoxins are at risk for developing a secondary malignancy such as AML (Pui et al., 1995).

Classifying AML using morphologic and cytogenic characteristics along with cell surface and biochemical markers is important (Wiley, 1993). The FAB Cooperative Group set up the most comprehensive system, which divides AML into seven subtypes: M1 through M7 (see Table 3-3). All FAB subtypes are represented in childhood and adolescent AML, although M6 AML is rare (Golub et al., 1997). M0, used to describe AML without localized differentiation, is not yet an official subtype. Special histochemical stains performed on bone marrow (e.g., myeloperoxidase, periodic acid-schiff, Sudan black B, esterase) will distinguish AML from other leukemia types. Further identification of cell surface and biochemical markers strengthens the histologic diagnosis of AML (Ebb & Weinstein, 1997). Immunophenotyping and chromosomal analysis yield important diagnostic information (Rubnitz & Look, 1998). Improved cytogenetic techniques such as FISH are helping to identify the multiple chromosomal abnormalities that are present in patients with AML.

Clinical Presentation of Acute Myelogenous Leukemia

Children with AML exhibit symptoms caused by bone marrow dysfunction. As a result of neutropenia, these children can present with complaints of fever and sore throat or other respiratory symptoms and persistent or recurrent bacterial infections. Anemia can cause pallor, weakness, fatigue, congestive heart failure, dyspnea, and headache. Bleeding, petechiae, bruising, epistaxis, and gingival oozing are the common signs of thrombocytopenia. Disseminated intravascular coagulation (DIC) also can cause bleeding and can occur in any FABG subtype, but it is particularly common in M3 as a result of an abnormal coagulation process (Golub et al., 1997; Wiley, 1993).

The total white blood cell count can range from normal to greater than 100,000 cells. Approximately 25% of children present with white blood cell counts greater than 100,000 cells (Golub et al., 1997). The absolute neutrophil count is usually depressed. Approximately 50% of newly diagnosed children have a platelet count less than 50,000. Hepatomegaly or splenomegaly is common. Significant lymphadenopathy is present in less than 25% of patients (Golub et al.). Chloromas—discrete tumors found in patients with AML—may develop in bones or soft tissues and can be seen in the epidural area and around the orbits. Extramedullary AML can invade the meninges, brain parenchyma, ovaries, or skin (leukemia cutis) and, rarely, the testes (Ebb & Weinstein, 1997). Central nervous system disease is present at diagnosis in a higher percentage of children with AML than those with ALL (Golub et al.). As with all types of leukemia, a thorough bone marrow analysis leads to the definitive diagnosis. AML is diagnosed when the bone marrow has more than 30% blasts with the characteristics of one of the FAB subdivisions of AML. The biopsy of a chloroma also can lead to the diagnosis.

Table 3-3. French-American-British Cooperative Group (FABCG) Classification of Acute Myelogenous Leukemia

FABCG Type	Common Name	Criteria for Diagnosis	Histochemistry
M1	Acute myeloblastic leukemia without maturation	• Blasts > 90% of nonerythroid cells • 10% of cells are maturing granulocytic or monocytes.	Myeloperoxidase (MP)+
M2	Acute myeloblastic leukemia with maturation	• Blasts from 30%–89% of nonerythroid cells • > 10% maturing granulocytic cells • < 20% monocytic cells	MP+
M3	Acute promyelocytic leukemia (hypergranular variant)	• < 20% abnormal hypergranular promyelocytes • Auer rods common	MP+
M3V	Acute promyelocytic leukemia (microgranular variant)	• Fine granular cytoplasm in promyelocytes • Nuclei may be reniform. • Electron microscopy shows multiple dark primary granules.	MP+
M4	Acute myelomonocytic leukemia	• Blasts > 30% of nonerythroid cells • > 20% but < 80% of cells are monocytic lineage. • Blood monocyte count > 5 x 10^6/l or elevated serum lysozyme level	MP+ Nonspecific esterase (NSE)+
M4Eo	Acute myelomonocytic leukemia with eosinophilia	• Abnormal eosinophils with specific eosinophilic granules and large basophilic granules	MP+ NSE+ Eos-periodic acid-Schiff (PAS)+
M5	Acute monocytic leukemia	• > 80% of nonerythroid cells are monoblasts, promonocytes, or monocytes. • M5a: > 80% of monocytic cells are monoblasts; M5b: < 80% of monocytic cells are monoblasts.	NSE+
M6	Erythroleukemia	• > 30% of nonerythroid cells are blasts, but > 50% of marrow cells are erythroblasts.	Erythroblasts PAS+
M7	Acute megakaryocytic leukemia	• >30% of nonerythroid cells are megakaryoblasts, cytoplasmic blebs, myelofibrosis.	Platelet perox + (EM)

Note. From "Acute Myelogenous Leukemia" (p. 465) by T.R. Golub, H.J. Weinstein, and H.E. Grier in P.A. Pizzo and D.G. Poplack (Eds.), *Principles and Practice of Pediatric Oncology* (3rd ed.), 1997, Philadelphia: Lippincott-Raven Publishers. Copyright 1997 by Lippincott-Raven Publishers. Reprinted with permission.

Very few consistent prognostic indicators have been identified with AML. In general, if patients present with a high white blood cell count (>100,000) or a secondary AML, have been treated for a myelodysplastic syndrome, or have a monosomy 7 karyotype, the remission rate is lower (Golub et al., 1997). Certain chromosome abnormalities such as +(8,21) have been connected with good remission rates as well as the ability to achieve a remission after one cycle (Grimwade et al., 1998). Possible adverse factors include the FABCG subtype M4 or M5, age (older or younger), splenomegaly, and M1 subtype with Auer rods—rod-shaped structures present in the cytoplasm that are pathognomic of leukemia (Ebb & Weinstein, 1997; Golub et al.). Children with Down syndrome have an increased risk of developing leukemia—predominantly AML—in the first three years. However, many children with Down syndrome who develop AML can be cured (Ravindranath et al., 1992).

Treatment Interventions for Children With Acute Myelogenous Leukemia

The treatment of AML involves the use of combination chemotherapy to control bone marrow and systemic disease. Intense treatment of the central nervous system is a standard part of most treatment protocols and is accomplished through the use of intrathecal chemotherapy, with or without cranial irradiation (Hurwitz et al., 1995; Wells et al., 1994).

Inducing a complete remission, which is defined by return of the marrow to a normal number of immature cells (< 5% myeloblasts), return of normal peripheral blood counts, and the resolution of extramedullary leukemic infiltration (i.e., lymphadenopathy), is the initial step required to prolong survival for patients with AML (Golub et al., 1997). Postremission consolidation or postremission intensification follows, with the goal of preventing recurrence. High-risk patients or those who relapse during therapy or shortly after may undergo bone marrow or stem cell transplantation as soon as the first remission is achieved (Ravindranath et al., 1996).

The induction phase of therapy is extremely intense. Two to three drugs are administered at very high doses for approximately six to eight months. The most common drugs administered are cytarabine, an anthracycline (usually daunomycin), and etoposide (VP16). The aim is to induce bone marrow aplasia. As a result, bleeding, infection, tumor lysis syndrome, and leukostasis all can present life-threatening situations (Ebb & Weinstein, 1997; Golub et al., 1997). Comprehensive supportive care (i.e., skilled nursing care, antibiotic therapy, blood and platelet transfusions, nutritional supplements, and psychological support) can decrease the mortality rate and improve patients' quality of life during this time (Ebb & Weinstein; Wells et al., 1994). Measures to help to shorten the duration of neutropenia range from the addition of hematopoietic growth factors, such as G-CSF, to induction therapy.

All patients with AML should undergo intensive remission induction. If stem cell or bone marrow transplantation is not planned, they should undergo further intensive therapy when in remission (Golub et al., 1997; Ravindranath et al., 1996). A third phase of therapy—maintenance chemotherapy—has not been proven to improve survival, especially for patients who have undergone very aggressive postremission therapy (Wells et al., 1994).

Two groups of patients with AML warrant specific attention. Patients with Down syndrome who develop AML tend to be younger, have either M6 or M7 subtypes, and have very good survival rates (Golub et al., 1997; Ravindranath et al., 1992), and patients who are diagnosed with acute promyelocytic leukemia (APL, FAB-M3) also warrant specific attention (see Table 3-3). Newly diagnosed patients who receive the combination of systemic chemotherapy and all-trans-retinoic acid

(ATRA) experience remission rates as high as 90% and a relapse-free survival rate of 70%–80% at two years (Golub et al.; Tallman et al., 1997).

Patients with recurrent or progressive AML have an overall dismal prognosis. Children or adolescents who relapse while not undergoing therapy have a higher chance of achieving a second remission (Golub et al., 1997). Autologous or allogeneic transplants during second or subsequent remissions offer a potential for long-term survival (Golub et al.; Petersen et al., 1993).

Although survival rates for AML have increased throughout the last 20 years, much research is aimed at drastically improving these numbers. Research involving the mechanism of leukemic cell differentiation, the use of growth factors to restore normal bone marrow function, and the process of drug resistance already has and will continue to alter therapeutic approaches to AML (Golub et al., 1997; Wells et al., 1994).

Central Nervous System Tumors

Overview

Primary brain tumors are the most common solid tumors occurring in children. Brain tumors are second to leukemia among all childhood cancers. Approximately 2.8 cases per 100,000 children are diagnosed per year (Gurney, Severson, Davis, & Robison, 1995). Central nervous system tumors rank high as a cause of mortality (Pollack, 1994). A small incidence peak of 2.2–2.5 cases per 100,000 children per year exists, with a slight male-to-female predominance (1.1:1) during the first decade of life. Within the first 10 years, embryonal neoplasms are predominant and the number of gliomas is low. This pattern continues into early adolescence, when the occurrence of supratentorial glial tumors increases. These tumors are typically adult central nervous system neoplasms (Heideman, Packer, Albright, Freeman, & Rorke, 1997).

Etiologic Factors Associated With Central Nervous System Tumors in Children and Adolescents

Central nervous system tumors and inherited syndromes are associated with each other. The association between neurofibromatosis and the development of low-grade optic gliomas, other glial tumors, and meningiomas is well-documented. Glial tumors and, occasionally, ependymomas are associated with tuberous sclerosis, and astrocytomas are linked with Li-Fraumeni syndrome and other pediatric solid tumors. Familial clusters of astrocytomas and glioblastoma multiforme have been reported to occur among siblings and other close relatives. Medulloblastomas occur in monozygotic twins, nontwin siblings, and patients with Turcot and ataxia-telangiectasia syndromes (Pollack, 1994; Prados et al., 1998).

Certain industrial and chemical toxins have been implicated in the development of central nervous system tumors. Reports of increased incidence in the children of parents who work with toxic agents are being evaluated. Some organic compounds (e.g., nitrous ureas, triazines, polycyclic hydrocarbons) are known central nervous system carcinogens in animals (Cohen & Duffman, 1994). Ionizing irradiation is associated with the development of brain tumors, and the occurrence of second malignancies after cranial irradiation in children has been documented (Furuta, Sugiu, Tamiya, Matsumoto, & Ohmoto, 1998).

The diagnosis of a brain tumor includes many histologic categories. Each is distinct in respect to the pathologic diagnosis and grade, ability to disseminate within and outside the central nervous system, clinical presentation, specific treatment, and overall prognosis. Table 3-4 provides a comparison of four morphologic classification systems. Bailey and Cushing established the first and most widely accepted system, which classified tumors based on morphology and presumed histogenesis. The most current classifications, Russell and Rubinstein and the World Health Organization (WHO) (which is modified for pediatrics in Table 3-4), are based on the earliest system. Russell and Rubinstein's system is based on their concepts of histogenesis, and the WHO system uses traditional morphologic entities, degree of anaplasia, and location within the central nervous system (Heideman et al., 1997). Only a modified form of the grading system for astrocytomas from the Kernohan and Associates system remains in use.

Pediatric brain tumors differ from adult brain tumors. Histologically, pediatric tumors have a wide range of features. Glial tumors are the most common histologic type occurring during childhood and adolescence. Of the most common tumors, approximately 25%–40% are supratentorial astrocytomas, 10%–20% cerebellar astrocytomas, 10%–20% medulloblastoma, 10%–20% brain stem gliomas, 6%–9% craniopharyngiomas, 5%–10% ependymoma, and 12%–14% other less common types (see Figure 3-1). More than half of these tumors are highly malignant. Pediatric tumors also differ by location. The majority of the pediatric tumors develop in the posterior fossa, and 75% of adult tumors are located supratentorially.

Clinical Presentation of Central Nervous System Tumors in Children and Adolescents

The clinical presentation varies with each child and depends on the tumor's location. The majority of pediatric brain tumors are in the posterior fossa, so the most frequent symptoms are related to increased intracranial pressure and hydrocephalus. These symptoms can include headache (usually worse in the morning), vomiting, irritability, apathy, and lethargy. As the intracranial pressure increases, it causes drowsiness that progresses to coma and depression of cardiac and respiratory function. Double vision, dysconjugate eye movements, papilledema, optic atrophy, and degrees of visual loss may occur. Other symptoms are specific to tumor location. Cerebellar tumors can cause ataxia, nystagmus, head tilt, abnormal reflexes, and scanning speech. Brain stem tumors commonly cause multiple cranial nerve abnormalities. Supratentorial tumors can have a wide range of symptoms that depend on the involved hemisphere and the presence of hydrocephalus. Temporal lobe lesions can cause seizures, and temporoparietal lesions can cause aphasia. Frontal lobe lesions can produce personality changes, and occipital lesions can affect vision. Midline tumors (e.g., germ cell tumors) can cause multiple endocrine abnormalities (Heideman et al., 1997; Petriccione, 1993).

Diagnostic Workup for Children or Adolescents With a Central Nervous System Tumor

Children with a suspected central nervous system neoplasm must undergo a thorough physical and neurologic examination. A detailed health history is imperative. Diagnostic neuroimaging of the head must be performed if a tumor is suspected. MRI is the test of choice because of the sensitivity of the imaging, ease of obtaining multiplanar images, minimal risk of allergic reaction to the contrast

Table 3-4. Comparison of Classification Systems for Central Nervous System Tumors

World Health Organization (modified for pediatrics)	Russell and Rubinstein	Kernohan and Associates	Bailey and Cushing
Glial Tumors	**Tumors of Glial Series**		
1. Astrocytic astrocytoma Anaplastic astrocytoma Subependymal giant cell tumor Giagnatocellular glioma	I. Astrocytic astrocytoma Astroblastoma	1. Astrocytoma grades I–IV	1. Astrocytoma 2. Astroblastoma
2. Oligodendroglial tumors Oligodendroglioma Anaplastic oligodendroglioma	II. Oligodendroglial tumors Oligodendroglioma	2. Oligodendroglioma grades I–IV	3. Oligodendroglioma
3. Ependymal tumors Ependymoma Anaplastic ependymoma Myxopapillary ependymoma	III. Tumors of the ependyma and its homologs Ependymoma	3. Ependymoma grades I–IV	4. Ependymoma 5. Ependymoblastoma
4. Choroid plexus tumors Choroid plexus papilloma Anaplastic choroid plexus tumor	Colloid cyst Choroid plexus papilloma		6. Choroid plexus papillomas
5. Mixed gliomas 6. Glioblastoma multiforme	IV. Glioblastoma multiforme	(Astrocytoma IV)	7. Glioblastoma multiforme
Neuronal Tumors	**Tumors of the Neuron Series**		
1. Gangliocytoma 2. Ganglioglioma 3. Anaplastic ganglioglioma	1. Ganglioneuroma 2. Ganglioglioma 3. Neuroblastoma	4. Neuroastrocytoma grades I–IV	8. Ganglioglioma 9. Neuroblastoma
Primitive Neuroectodermal Tumors (PNET)			
1. PNET not otherwise specified 2. PNET with differentiation (astrocytic, ependymal, neuronal); oligodendroglial, mixed	4. Medulloblastoma	5. Medulloblastoma	10. Medulloblastoma
3. Medulloepithelioma	5. Medulloepithelioma	(Ependymoma IV)	11. Medulloepithelioma
Pineal Cell Tumors	**Pineal Parenchymal Tumors**		
1. Pineocytoma 2. PNET (pineoblastoma)	1. Pineocytoma 2. Pineoblastoma		12. Pinealoma

Note. From "Tumors of the Central Nervous System" (p. 637) by R.L. Heideman, R.J. Packer, L.A. Albright, C.R. Freeman, and L.B. Rorke in P.A. Pizzo and D.G. Poplack (Eds.) *Principles and Practice of Pediatric Oncology* (3rd ed.), 1997, Philadelphia: Lippincott-Raven Publishers. Copyright 1997 by Lippincott-Raven Publishers. Reprinted with permission.

Figure 3-1. Most Commonly Occurring Pediatric Brain Tumors

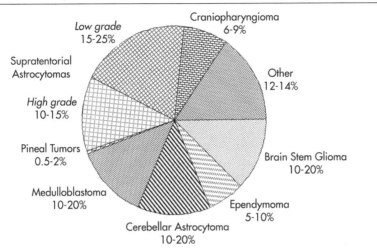

Note. From "Tumors of the Central Nervous System" (p. 634) by R.L. Heideman, R.J. Packer, L.A. Albright, C.R. Freeman, and L.B. Rorke in P.A. Pizzo and D.G. Poplack (Eds.) *Principles and Practice of Pediatric Oncology* (3rd. ed.), 1997, Philadelphia: Lippincott-Raven Publishers. Copyright 1997 by Lippincott-Raven Publishers. Reprinted with permission.

medium gadolinium, and lack of radiation exposure (Prados et al., 1998). If MRI is not available immediately, a CT scan, with and without iodinated contrast, should be performed. MRI of the spine is performed if disease symptoms are present or if tumors that are known to disseminate to the spinal cord are present. A lumbar puncture may be performed to determine the presence of disease in the cerebrospinal fluid, indicating dissemination throughout the neuraxis, or to look for tumor "markers" as in germ cell tumors. A bone marrow aspirate and biopsy also may be performed in cases where systemic dissemination in suspected (Cohen & Duffman, 1994). Other neuroimaging techniques can be used initially or as treatment progresses to evaluate response. PET is a sensitive diagnostic test especially useful in assessing recurrent tumors. PET can measure metabolic activity and distinguish between malignancy (which presents as hypermetabolism) and radiation-injured or necrotic brain (which presents as reduced metabolism) (Prados et al.). To further help to differentiate active tumor from injured brain, MRS can be used with MRI to evaluate amounts of certain phosphorous-containing compounds. Function MRI can help to facilitate surgical planning by pinpointing critical areas of function in the brain of specific patients (Heideman et al., 1997).

Treatment Interventions for Children or Adolescents With a Central Nervous System Tumor

In most cases, once a tumor has been imaged, surgery is the next step. The goal is to obtain the most complete resection possible while preserving neurologic function. At the very least, a biopsy should be performed to determine pathology. Stereotactic procedures now make obtaining tissue from almost all brain areas possible (Prados et al., 1998). One notable exception is the "classic" diffuse pontine brain stem lesion. The surgical procedure used to obtain tissue from this area can cause harm without significantly altering the prognosis. Another exception involves certain germ cell tumors that can be diagnosed by the presence of specific tumor markers. Many things should be considered when planning a surgical procedure. A complete resection of a low-grade tumor such as a juvenile pilocytic astrocytoma will result in a "cure" with no further therapy. When a complete resection is not an option, performing the most extensive resection possible is advantageous for obvious reasons (Youmans, 1996). A tumor that is causing symptoms as a result of increased pressure will clinically improve. In most cases, when determining the pathology, studying a large sampling of the tumor is more accurate because "sampling errors" can be avoided. In primary central nervous system lymphoma, however, a biopsy alone will establish an accurate diagnosis (Heideman et al., 1997). With this diagnosis, tumor resection does not affect the prognosis. With certain brain tumor types (e.g., anaplastic astrocytomas), the degree of the original resection does affect prognosis. The exact mechanism is unknown, but follow-up therapy perhaps is more effective when less tumor burden exists. Intricate surgical procedures using previously described imaging techniques make the debulking of larger tumors with less morbidity more feasible (Sawaya et al., 1998; Youmans).

Radiation therapy for central nervous system tumors usually is administered using x-rays, gamma rays, neutrons, protons, and other heavy particles, with DNA damage being the major event in tumor cell destruction (Heideman et al., 1997). This therapy has been crucial in the treatment of all brain tumors that are not surgically curable. CT and MRI are used to plan individual radiation treatment courses by determining tumor pathology, the potential to disseminate throughout the neuraxis, location, and size of the lesion. Children's age also is a factor in planning radiation treatment courses. Precision is crucial in the delivery of focal doses of irradiation or dosage boosts to the primary area so that only the targeted areas of the brain are affected. The usual treatment course is approximately six weeks, with daily treatments administered five consecutive days each week. Standard treatment for brain tumors that can disseminate throughout the central nervous system (e.g., medulloblastoma) is 3,500–4,500 centigray (cGy) to the neuraxis, with a posterior fossa boost to 5,500 cGy total. Lower doses may be administered to the spinal cord in protocols that combine intensive chemotherapy (Deutsch et al., 1996). High focal doses of 5,500–6,000 cGy are administered to the primary tumor site of certain lesions (e.g., high-grade astrocytomas). Interstitial brachytherapy is another approach used in local tumor control. Temporary implants that deliver additional focal irradiation during a four- to five-day period are placed using stereotactic procedures (Youmans, 1996). The risk of developing necrosis in the tumor bed and surrounding areas is significant. A second similar option is to have implants placed during the initial resection that deliver lower doses of irradiation per day during a longer time period. This approach appears to have a lower risk of necrosis when treating larger tumor areas (Halligan et al., 1996). Radiosurgery (e.g., surgery performed with a gamma knife) has been successful with local control of small, deep malignant tumors (Heideman et al.). A gamma knife is a gamma irradiation device that delivers a focused radiation beam to a tumor target in the brain.

Radiation therapy has a broad range of sequelae. Although the majority of children and adolescents tolerate the treatment well, an increase in cerebral edema can cause headache and vomiting. Dexamethasone can minimize this effect. Alopecia, erythema of the skin, otitis externa or secretory otitis media, ear pain, tinnitus, and mild hearing loss are all transient early problems that usually require only symptomatic treatment. Transient hematologic suppression can be experienced with irradiation to the brain and spinal cord. Approximately six to eight weeks after the completion of treatment, temporary demyelination may cause the "somnolence syndrome." This usually lasts for approximately two weeks. The complaints related to this syndrome are lethargy, anorexia, headache, and vomiting. Although the syndrome resolves completely without sequelae, low-dose steroids can give symptomatic relief (Petriccione, 1993). Delayed radiation-induced damage can range from neuropsychological disabilities to tissue necrosis (Moore, 1995). The development of secondary central nervous system tumors also has been documented (Furuta et al., 1998). Children under three years of age suffer devastating sequelae when treated with radiation therapy to the central nervous system. The toxicities include growth failure, mental retardation, and leukoencephalopathy. These children now are treated first with intensive chemotherapy in an effort to delay or eliminate the need for this therapy (Duffner et al., 1993).

Multiple studies conducted by the major cooperative study groups (e.g., CCG, POG) have proven the efficacy of chemotherapy. Chemotherapy is usually part of a multifaceted treatment protocol and can be administered before, during, and after radiation therapy and as an alternative to radiation therapy in the case of very young children. Advances in methods of administration, dosing, and sequence of chemotherapeutic agents have been made (Ater, 1998). The most commonly administered chemotherapeutic drugs are alkylating agents used as single agents or in combination with other drugs (Prados & Russo, 1998). High-dose chemotherapy followed by autologous bone marrow transplantation or peripheral blood stem cell reinfusion has been successful in treating malignant, chemosensitive tumors such as medulloblastoma (Kedar et al., 1994). This allows higher doses to be administered safely because the duration of pancytopenia is shortened. As previously discussed, chemotherapy now is used to treat young children as an initial line of therapy with the goal being to avoid or, at the very least, delay radiation therapy until they are older (Duffner et al., 1993; Giordana, Schiffer, & Schiffer, 1998). Recurrent or progressive disease also can be treated with intensive chemotherapy protocols followed by peripheral blood stem cell rescues (Graham et al., 1997; Heideman et al., 1997). Single agents, such as oral etoposide, are under evaluation in progressive disease (Needle et al., 1997).

A brief description of the management of three different types of brain tumors will help to illustrate the various therapeutic strategies that can be utilized.

Medulloblastoma/Primitive Neuroectodermal Tumors

Histologically, primitive neuroectodermal tumors (PNETs) can show areas of glial, neuronal, or ependymal differentiation or can be undifferentiated. Isochromosome 17q is the most common cytogenic abnormality (Giordana et al., 1998). They can develop in many areas: lesions in the cerebellum are called medulloblastomas, lesions in the pineal region of the brain are called pinealoblastomas, and lesions in the cerebrum are called cerebral PNETs (Prados et al., 1998). These tumors can disseminate throughout the central nervous system and, occasionally, to bone, lungs, and other organs (Scheurlen & Kuhl, 1998). Two broad classifications are used to determine treatment plans. Average- or standard-risk patients are defined as children older than three years with posterior fossa tumors, complete or "near-complete" resection (< 1.5 cc of residual disease), and no dissemination. Poor- or high-risk patients are defined as children younger than three years with subtotal resections (> 1.5 cc of residual disease) and disseminated disease or nonposterior fossa location.

Average-risk patients are treated with surgery, irradiation, and chemotherapy, which usually is administered during and following radiation treatment. The goal of this regimen is to reduce the dose of the radiation therapy, and researchers continue to evaluate this possibility (Kuhl, 1998). Approximately 75% of these patients are disease free at five years. Poor-risk patients have a 35%–50% chance of disease-free survival at five years. More intensive chemotherapy has increased the survival rate in this group as high as 60% in some studies. Children younger than age three undergo intensive chemotherapy without radiation therapy (Dunkel & Finlay, 1996). Children with recurrent disease are treated aggressively with high-dose chemotherapy followed by an autologous stem cell rescue (Dunkel et al., 1998). Intensive chemotherapy has significantly affected disease control in this group.

Ependymoma

Ependymomas are derived from ependymal cells, with 25%–40% developing above the tentorium and 60%–75% developing below the tentorium. Approximately 10% of ependymomas develop in the spinal cord. The SV40 polyomavirus and related polyomaviruses can induce ependymoma and choroid plexus tumors in monkeys (Heideman et al., 1997). These viruses belong to the papovirus family, a strain that is important in viral investigations of carcinogenesis. Ependymomas are invasive tumors that spread into adjacent brain tissue. They rarely metastasize, but they can spread to the liver, lungs, and bone. The degree of resection is crucial with this tumor and may be the single most important prognostic factor (Heideman et al.). Invasion of the brain stem and young age (particularly younger than five to seven years) are poor prognostic factors. Overall, patients with spinal cord ependymomas are a distinct entity. The myxopapillary ependymoma of the cauda equina has a better prognosis. No recognized grading system exists, but tumors with anaplastic features are considered high-grade. Tumors that develop within the ventricle have a higher tendency to spread throughout the subarachnoid space, resulting in disseminated disease. Workup should include an MRI of the spine and examination of cerebrospinal fluid for cytology (Bouffet, Perilongo, Canete, & Massimimo, 1998; Robertson et al., 1998). Radiation therapy should be administered to the posterior fossa to treat infratentorial ependymomas. With metastasis to the cerebrospinal fluid, craniospinal irradiation is administered. Craniospinal irradiation also may be administered to treat anaplastic tumors, which are high-grade tumors. Focal irradiation therapy should be administered to the tumor area to treat supratentorial ependymomas. Administering craniospinal irradiation to the more anaplastic tumors or those adjacent to the ventricular lining when no dissemination is documented is controversial (McLaughlin et al., 1998). The role of adjuvant chemotherapy continues to be investigated. Children under three years of age undergo chemotherapy to avoid irradiation (Duffner et al., 1993; Mason et al., 1998). Chemotherapy also is used to treat recurrent disease after surgical options are explored.

Brain Stem Glioma

Brain stem gliomas occur more frequently in young children and can develop in the midbrain, pons, and medulla oblongata. Diffuse intrinsic tumors, usually developing in the pons, account for approximately 80% of all these tumors (Heideman et al., 1997). These tumors are not surgically accessible but may be biopsied if exophytic extension is present, meaning the tumor extends beyond the brain stem. Radiation therapy initially may have a therapeutic effect, but rapid tumor progression is usual, with a median survival rate of less than one year (Freeman & Farmer, 1998). The other subclassifications include focal, cystic, dorsal exophytic, and cervicomedullary. Prognosis differs among each type and depends on location, histologic features, surgical access, and degree of resection. Some patients with small focal tumors may have a good prognosis with surgery alone. Radiation therapy is administered to all patients with high-grade disease, progressive disease, or surgically inaccessible disease (Freeman & Farmer). Chemotherapy has not been effective with this disease, although some single agents have shown limited antitumor activity with recurrence. As with other brain tumors, children under three years of age may undergo chemotherapy in an effort to delay radiation therapy (Mason et al., 1998).

Future Considerations

Significant advances have been made with the treatment of certain types of brain tumors, particularly those that are surgically resectable. The increased use of chemotherapy in many treatment protocols has drastically increased the overall prognosis, especially with tumors such as medulloblastoma that are known to metastasize within and beyond the central nervous system. The increased sophistication of imaging, surgical procedures, and the ability to deliver radiation therapy has improved not only survival rates but also the quality of life of the survivors.

Laboratory and clinical research has increased in the area of central nervous system tumors throughout the last decade. Research is ongoing in many areas. New agents, mechanisms of resistance to standard chemotherapeutic agents, inhibitors of growth factors and their receptors, angiogenesis, and gene therapy are being studied (Prados et al., 1998). Children and adolescents with central nervous system tumors present special challenges that result from the tumor, treatment, and side effects. A multidisciplinary team must care for these children and adolescents, monitoring all aspects of therapy throughout their life span (Jenkin, 1996). Ongoing research is focused not only on specific treatment protocols for the various brain tumors but also on addressing issues such as neurocognitive impairment that directly impact the quality of life of brain tumor survivors.

Non-Hodgkin's Lymphoma

Overview

Approximately 500 new cases of NHL, the third most common malignancy found in children and adolescents, are diagnosed each year in the United States (Robinson, 1997; Sandlund, Downing, & Crist, 1996). It can be diagnosed at any time from infancy through young adulthood, although it is most common between 10 and 20 years of age. Statistically, it occurs twice as often among the white population as it does among blacks and approximately three times as often among boys than among girls (Sandlund et al., 1996).

The exact cause of this disease is unknown, although occupational and environmental exposures, genetics, and immunologic and viral agents are associated with its development (Skarin & Dorfman, 1997). High-risk children or adolescents are those with AIDS or a congenital immunodeficiency (e.g., ataxia-telangiectasia), those who have undergone chemotherapy or radiotherapy for a previous neoplasm, and organ recipients (McClain, Joshi, & Murphy, 1996; Sandlund et al., 1996; Taylor, Metcalfe, Thick, & Mak, 1996). Deficient T cell function is believed to be partially responsible for this increased risk (Sandlund et al., 1996). EBV may have a role in the development of Burkitt's lymphoma. EBV is associated with the development of NHL in African children and also has been found in sporadic cases in the United States and in South America (Beral & Newton, 1998; Razzouk, Srinivas, Sample, Singh, & Sixbey, 1996; Shad & Magrath, 1997). The histologic classification of NHL can be divided into three broad categories: lymphoblastic lymphoma, small noncleaved cell lymphoma (Burkitt's and non-Burkitt's), and large-cell lymphoma. Each category then is divided further on the basis of histology, phenotype, or a combination of both. The primary disease site varies according to the histologic subtype (see Table 3-5).

Lymphoblastic lymphoma comprises approximately 30% of all childhood NHL. Approximately 95% of lymphoblastic lymphomas are derived from immature T cells and express several distinct phenotypic markers, such as the enzyme terminal deoxynucleotidyl transferase (TdT) (Sandlund et al., 1996). A small percentage are precursors B cell type (Skarin & Dorfman, 1997). The malignant cells are small to intermediate in size with distinct nuclear membranes, inconspicuous nucleoli, fine chromatin, and a small rim of cytoplasm (Sandlund et al., 1996; Skarin & Dorfman).

Small noncleaved cell lymphomas comprise approximately 40%–50% of all childhood NHL and include Burkitt's and non-Burkitt's types. These lymphomas are of B cell origin, lack TdT, and, in almost all cases, express cALLa (CD10), which is a cell surface antigen (Sandlund et al., 1996). The tumors pathologically show sheets of lymphoid cells with prominent nucleoli and a distinct rim of basophilic cytoplasm. Normal macrophages scattered throughout the tumor cause a classic "starry sky" appearance (Shad & Magrath, 1997).

Large-cell lymphoma comprises approximately 20%–25% of all childhood NHL. These tumors can have either a B or T cell lineage, which are the major types, or they can be of indeterminate lineage (Murphy, Fairclough, Hutchison, & Berard, 1989; Shad & Magrath, 1997). In children, these immunophenotypes occur with approximately equal frequency. The anaplastic large-cell lymphoma is predominantly of T cell lineage and contains large, "bizarre-appearing" cells with abundant cytoplasm, irregular nuclei, and prominent nucleoli in sheets of adherent cells (Sandlund et al., 1994). B cell large-cell lymphoma may present clinically similar to the small noncleaved lymphomas, although they present more often as a localized disease. B cell large-cell lymphoma shares similar immunophenotyping and chromosomal abnormalities (Hutchinson et al., 1998). In general, the large-cell lymphomas that lack evidence of either T or B cell lineage behave clinically like the T cell large-cell lymphomas (Shad & Magrath).

Pretreatment staging of this disease is crucial. The criteria outlined in Table 3-6 determine pretreatment staging. The main clinical staging systems that are used also are summarized in Table

Table 3-5. Clinical and Biologic Characteristics of Non-Hodgkin's Lymphoma in Children

Subtype[a]	Proportion of Cases (%)[b]	Phenotype	Primary Site
Small noncleaved cell (Burkitt's)	34	B cell	Abdomen or head and neck
Lymphoblastic	29	T cell[c]	Mediastinum or head and neck
Large cell	27	B cell, T cell inde-terminate	Mediastinum, abdomen, head and neck, or skin

[a] The subtypes are classified according to the National Cancer Institute's working formulation.
[b] Other histologic subtypes account for approximately 10% of cases.
[c] B cell progenitor variants also have been described.

Note. From "Non-Hodgkin's Lymphoma in Childhood," by J.T. Sandlund, J.R. Downing, and W.M. Christ, 1996, *New England Journal of Medicine, 334,* p. 1239. Copyright 1996 by the Massachusetts Medical Society. Reprinted with permission.

3-6. The accuracy of staging is important because of the distinct differences in the intensity and duration of therapy and the prognosis of patients with limited (stage I or II) and advanced disease (stage III or IV) (Sandlund et al., 1996). With stage IV disease, an arbitrary distinction is made with the extent of bone marrow involvement. Patients who have more than 25% of their bone marrow replaced with tumor cells are diagnosed with acute lymphoblastic leukemia or leukemia/lymphoma (Sandlund et al., 1996). The histology and clinical stage together form the basis for the definitive diagnosis.

Diagnostic Workup for Children and Adolescents With Non-Hodgkin's Lymphoma

A detailed health history encompassing prior history and the present concerns must accompany a thorough, comprehensive physical examination. The diagnostic workup then is planned in an accurate and timely fashion to ensure that treatment begins as quickly as possible. The following studies are performed: (a) standard blood tests including a complete blood count, differential blood count, examination of the blood smear, LDH, Bg-microglobulin levels, liver function tests, renal function tests, serum electrolytes, calcium, and uric acid levels, (b) bilateral bone marrow aspirates and biopsies, (c) lumbar puncture and evaluation of spinal fluid, and (d) radiologic studies including chest x-ray (posteroanterior and lateral views), chest CT scan if the chest x-ray is abnormal or respiratory symptoms are present, abdomen and pelvic CT scan, and a gallium-G7 scan, which is particularly important with high-grade lymphomas. Studies that are tailored to further evaluate a specific symptom could include a CT scan or MRI (preferably) of the head and spine to address cranial/spinal complaints, upper and lower gastrointestinal tract contrast studies or ultrasound for abdominal problems, and a tectinietium 99 scan, commonly known as a bone scan, or bone x-rays to address skeletal complaints (Shad & Magrath, 1997; Skarin & Dorfman, 1997).

Clinical Presentation of Children and Adolescents With Non-Hodgkin's Lymphoma

Almost two-thirds of adolescents with NHL present with locally advanced disease or metastatic disease (Sandlund et al., 1996). The disease history is usually short with rapid progression of symptoms. The specific clinical complaints depend on the histologic type, the stage of disease, and the tumor's primary location (Sandlund et al., 1996; Shad & Magrath, 1997). Children and adolescents typically have extranodal disease involving the mediastinum (26% of cases), abdomen (31% of cases), or head and neck (29% of cases) (Sandlund et al., 1996; Shad & Magrath). Approximately 75% of patients with lymphoblastic lymphoma present with an anterior mediastinal mass that may have an associated pleural effusion, stridor, dyspnea, dysphasia, or head and neck swelling. As many as 90% of patients with small noncleaved cell lymphoma present with intra-abdominal tumors that can cause pain, nausea, vomiting, and distension. Patients with large abdominal masses are at risk for tumor lysis syndrome at the start of chemotherapy and will need vigorous hydration, alkalinization, and the administration of allopurinol or urate oxidase (Sandlund et al., 1996; Shad & Magrath). Dissemination of the disease may present as pancytopenia, indicative of advanced disease. Large-cell lymphoma may present with an anterior mediastinal mass or abdominal disease, although it is most often localized and less often invades the bone marrow or central nervous system (Sandlund et al., 1996; Shad & Magrath).

Table 3-6. Clinical Staging Systems for Childhood Lymphomas

Stage	Memorial Sloan-Kettering Cancer Center	St. Jude Children's Research Hospital	Stage	National Cancer Institute
I	One single site	Single tumor (extranodal) or single anatomic area (nodal) with the exclusion of mediastinum or abdomen	A	Single solitary extra-abdominal site
II	Two or more sites on same side of diaphragm	Single tumor (extranodal) with regional node involvement Two or more nodal areas on the same side of the diaphragm Two single (extranodal) tumors, with or without regional node involvement, on the same side of the diaphragm Primary gastrointestinal tract tumor, usually in the ileocecal area, with or without involvement of associated mesenteric nodes only	B	Multiple extra-abdominal sites
III	Disseminated disease without marrow or central nervous system involvement	Two single tumors (extranodal) on opposite sides of the diaphragm Two or more nodal areas above and below the diaphragm All the primary intrathoracic tumors (mediastinal, pleural, thymic) All extensive primary intra-abdominal disease All paraspinal or epidural tumors, regardless of other tumor site	C	Intra-abdominal tumor
IV	Any of above with bone marrow and/or central nervous system involvement	Any of the above, with initial central nervous system or bone marrow involvement (< 25% blasts)	D	Intra-abdominal tumor with involvement of one or more extra-abdominal sites
IVA	Bone marrow with < 25% blasts		AR	Intra-abdominal tumor with more than 90% of tumor surgically resected
IVB	Bone marrow with > 25% blasts			

Note. From "Non-Hodgkin's Lymphoma" (p. 267) by Q.N. McGowan in G.V. Foley, D. Fochtman, and K.H. Mooney (Eds.) *Nursing Care of the Child With Cancer* (2nd ed.), 1993, Philadelphia: W.B. Saunders Co. Copyright 1993 by W.B. Saunders Co. Reprinted with permission.

Certain consistent clinical features are associated with prognostic outcome. The tumor burden, reflected by the stage of the disease and the serum LDH concentration, is most predictive of the outcome (Sandlund et al., 1996). Patients who present with central nervous system disease (in Burkitt's lymphoma) or bone marrow involvement appear to have a poorer prognosis. Some researchers believe that the expression of CD30 in adolescents with large-cell lymphomas may indicate a good prognosis, but it more commonly is thought that surface markers are not accurate prognostic indicators (Sandlund et al., 1994).

Treatment Interventions for Children and Adolescents With Non-Hodgkin's Lymphoma

Systemic treatment is the cornerstone of therapy for adolescents with NHL (Murphy et al., 1989). Other than for obtaining a biopsy, the benefits of surgical intervention are limited. With some specific cases, for example, completely removing a gastrointestinal tract tumor is possible, resulting in less intensive therapy. Irradiation is not used routinely as a treatment modality. It is usually restricted to emergency situations, for example, in which severe mass effect results in airway obstruction or evidence exists of central nervous system disease.

Multiagent chemotherapy protocols used to treat NHL differ in the selection of chemotherapeutic agents, schedule of treatments, and intensity and duration of the treatment schema. The histology and stage of the NHL determine the chemotherapy protocol that is used. To prevent spread to the central nervous system, intrathecal and high-dose chemotherapy are used, except in limited-stage disease with no head or neck involvement. If central nervous system disease is present at diagnosis, intensified combination intrathecal drugs are given and, except in Burkitt's lymphoma, cranial irradiation is added (Anderson et al., 1993; Reiter et al., 1995; Tubergen et al., 1995). Table 3-7 provides an overview of chemotherapeutic regimens and the percentage of long-term survival according to non-Hodgkin's lymphoma staging.

The prognosis is excellent for adolescents with stage I or II NHL of any histologic subtype. Patients with stage I or II Burkitt's or large-cell lymphoma can undergo successful therapy during a nine-week period, although this shortened treatment time remains controversial. With the shortened treatment period, overall survival rates were similar to those reported for children with other histologic lymphoma subtypes, but 33% of the children with lymphoblastic lymphoma required intensive therapy for relapsed or refractory disease (Link, Shuster, Donaldson, Berard, & Murphy, 1993; Sandlund et al., 1996).

Recent trials show that adolescents with advanced-stage Burkitt's lymphoma have a long-term survival rate of approximately 70%–80%. The most effective approach is very intensive therapy administered throughout a two- to eight-month period. Effective treatment protocols for advanced stage lymphoblastic NHL are derived from protocols that are used to treat acute lymphoblastic leukemia and use as many as 10 drugs in three phases: induction of remission, consolidation, and maintenance (Bowman et al., 1996; Tubergen et al., 1995). The optimal regimens are complex with a strong possibility of toxic side effects. Central nervous system prophylaxis should be given to all patients with disseminated disease even if the central nervous system disease cannot be detected. When the central nervous system is involved at diagnosis, irradiation should be considered (Bowman et al., 1996; Tubergen et al.). Stage III and IV large-cell NHL is difficult to treat because of its diverse biologic properties. Adolescents with B cell tumors respond well to short-term inten-

Table 3-7. Outcome of Stage-Directed Chemotherapy in Children With Non-Hodgkin's Lymphoma

| Stage | Chemotherapeutic Regimen | | Long Term Survival (%)* | Comments |
	Agents	Period		
I or II (limited)				
Burkitt's or large-cell lymphoma	Cyclophosphamide, vincristine, and prednisone, with or without doxorubicin or methotrexate	9–26 weeks	85–95	Expected late effects of therapy are minimal.
Lymphoblastic lymphoma	Cyclophosphamide, vincristine, and prednisone, with or without doxorubicin, methotrexate, mercaptopurine, asparaginase, thioguanine, cytarabine, or carmustine	33 weeks–24 months	85–90	With the shorter duration of therapy, retreatment is required in approximately one-third of cases.
III or IV (advanced)				
Burkitt's lymphoma	Cyclophosphamide, vincristine, prednisone, and high-dose methotrexate, with or without etoposide, ifosfamide, doxorubicin, cytarabine, or cisplatin	2–8 months	75–85	Relapses are rare more than one year after diagnosis.
Lymphoblastic lymphoma	Vincristine, prednisone, daunorubicin or doxorubicin, and asparaginase, with or without methotrexate, cytarabine, high-dose methotrexate, cyclophosphamide, mercaptopurine, thioguanine, teniposide, hydroxyurea, or carmustine	15–32 months	65–75	Relapses can occur as late as three years after diagnosis or, in rare cases, later.
Large-cell lymphoma	Vincristine, prednisone, and methotrexate with or without high-dose methotrexate, cyclophosphamide, mercaptopurine, thioguanine, hydroxyurea, asparaginase, daunorubicin or doxorubicin, carmustine, or bleomycin	3–24 months	50–70	Among the patients with relapses after therapy, the survival rate is approximately 40% with high-dose chemotherapy and autologous bone marrow transplantation.

[a] Estimates are for survival at three to five years without the need for retreatment (event-free survival). For limited-stage lymphoblastic disease, the estimates include event-free survival and successful treatment of refractory disease.

Note. From "Non-Hodgkin's Lymphoma in Childhood," by J.T. Sandlund, J.R. Downing, and W.M. Christ, 1996, *New England Journal of Medicine, 334,* p. 1888. Copyright 1996 by the Massachusetts Medical Society. Reprinted with permission.

sive regimens (used for Burkitt's lymphoma), while those with T cell tumors probably require more intensive, prolonged therapy (Sandlund et al., 1996).

In general, the prognosis for children or adolescents with relapsed disease is poor, especially if the initial therapy was appropriately intensive. Aggressive treatments are used to induce patients into second remissions, at which time an allogeneic or autologous bone marrow transplantation may be considered.

Future Research

Future efforts need to focus on the patients who present with advanced disease. More intensive therapeutic regimens may be administered with less toxic effects (e.g., the use of hematopoietic colony stimulating factors such as G-CSF, autologous transplantation of peripheral blood stem cells). As a more clear outline of clinical and biologic prognostic factors becomes available, targeting patients who require more aggressive initial treatment may become easier, thus reducing the number of treatment failures (Magrath et al., 1996).

Hodgkin's Disease

Overview

Hodgkin's disease is a lymphoma that is characterized by the presence of multinucleated giant cells called Reed-Sternberg cells. Three distinct forms of this disease exist: childhood (14 years of age and younger), young adult (15–34 years of age), and older adult (55–74 years of age). Age distribution is bimodal, with an early peak in the mid to late 20s and a second peak in later childhood. It is rare before five years of age. The incidence is higher in boys under the 10 years of age. In adolescents, the male-to-female ratio is fairly equal. Most older adolescents with Hodgkin's disease are white (Hudson & Donaldson, 1997). More than 90% of newly diagnosed children and adolescents will be cured (see Table 3-1).

Etiologic Factors Associated With Hodgkin's Disease in Children and Adolescents

The etiology of Hodgkin's disease is uncertain. Clustering of cases among close relatives, especially same-sex siblings, suggests a genetic predisposition (Hudson & Donaldson, 1997). The higher risk also may be associated with similar environmental exposures. This malignancy is one of the few in which familiar occurrences involving close relatives frequently revealed concordant human leukocyte antigen (HLA) typing (Hudson & Donaldson). Hodgkin's disease is more common in individuals with an immunodeficiency disease such as ataxia-telangiectasia. Infectious agents such as cytomegalovirus and EBV may be associated with Hodgkin's disease. In the United States, EBV is present in the Reed-Sternberg cells of approximately one-third of newly diagnosed cases (Jarret, Armstrong, & Alexander, 1996).

The currently used histologic classification system for childhood Hodgkin's disease is the Rye modification of the Lukes and Butler (1966) system. The four categories are lymphocyte predominance, nodular sclerosis, mixed cellularity, and lymphocyte depletion. Lymphocyte predominant

Hodgkin's disease is localized and appears to require less-intensive therapy. Nodular sclerosis Hodgkin's disease is the most common subtype and is especially prevalent in adolescents (approximately 70% of cases). The mixed cellularity subtype is more common in younger children (< 10 years of age) and frequently is associated with advanced disease. The lymphocyte depletion category is rare in children. Patients in this category usually have widespread disease at diagnosis. As a result of intensive multiagent treatment protocols, histologic subtype does not appear to affect prognosis (Shankar et al., 1997).

Staging determines the extent of disease present at diagnosis and is crucial in deciding the course of treatment that is needed. The Ann Arbor staging system currently is used for Hodgkin's disease. Table 3-8 describes each stage. Stages I, II, III, and IV can be subclassifed into A and B categories. "A" indicates asymptomatic patients, and "B" indicates patients with any of the following symptoms: unexplained fever with temperature above 38°C for more than three days, drenching night sweats, or unexplained weight loss (> 10% of body weight) during the six months prior to diagnosis. The subclassification "E" denotes minimal extralymphatic disease. In addition, a CS to indicate clinical staging or PS to indicate pathologic staging is assigned to each stage with a plus sign (+) and symbol for each site of extralymphatic involvement. The staging laparotomy yields the pathologic staging information (Hudson & Donaldson, 1997).

Clinical Presentation of Children or Adolescents With Hodgkin's Disease

Children with suspected Hodgkin's disease may present with a wide range of symptoms. The most common presenting sign is cervical or supraclavicular adenopathy with characteristically painless, firm, and movable lymph nodes. A mediastinal mass may accompany cervical adenopathy.

Table 3-8. Ann Arbor Staging Classification for Hodgkin's Disease

Stage	Definition
I	Involvement of a single lymph node region (I) or of a single extralymphatic organ or site (I_E)
II	Involvement of two or more lymph node regions on the same side of the diaphragm (II) or localized involvement of an extralymphatic organ or site and one or more lymph node regions on the same side of the diaphragm (II_E)
III	Involvement of lymph node regions on both sides of the diaphragm (III), which may be accompanied by involvement of the spleen (III_S) or by localized involvement of an extralymphatic organ or site (III_E) or both (III_{SE})
IV	Diffuse or disseminated involvement of one or more extralymphatic organs or tissues with or without associated lymph node involvement

Note. The absence or presence of fever over 38°C for three consecutive days, drenching night sweats, or unexplained loss of 10% or more of body weight in the six months preceding admission are to be denoted in all cases by the suffix letters A or B, respectively.

Note. From "Hodgkin's Disease" (p. 529) by M.H. Hudson and S.S. Donaldson in P.A. Pizzo and D.G. Poplack (Eds.) Principles and Practice of Pediatric Oncology (3rd ed.), 1997, Philadelphia: Lippincott-Raven Publishers. Copyright 1997 by Lippincott-Raven Publishers. Reprinted with permission.

The presence of organomegaly (spleen or liver) usually indicates widespread disease. Anorexia, slight weight loss, malaise, and lethargy are common in children. The presence of the "B" symptoms previously described has prognostic significance. Pruritus, a symptom more common in adults, does not have prognostic significance.

Diagnostic Workup for Children or Adolescents With Hodgkin's Disease

A thorough history and physical examination are performed with particular attention to the measurement of palpable adenopathy. Laboratory studies include a complete blood count, erythrocyte sedimentation rate, serum copper and iron levels, serum ferritin and transferrin determinations, renal and liver function tests, and baseline thyroid function tests. The presence of anemia may indicate advanced disease. The erythrocyte sedimentation rate, serum copper, and ferritin levels may be elevated, but they are not prognostically significant. Patients with Hodgkin's disease usually have immune system abnormalities characterized by altered T and B lymphocyte functioning. These abnormalities may persist during and after treatment (Hudson & Donaldson, 1997; Raney et al., 1997). A chest x-ray with anteroposterior and lateral views is performed. A biopsy of nodular tissue is performed to establish pathologic diagnosis. A CT of the chest, abdomen, and pelvis should be performed. A neck CT should be performed if high cervical adenopathy is present. A gallium scan is particularly useful in evaluating supradiaphragmatic disease. A bone marrow biopsy is performed for patients with clinical stage III or IV, who present with B symptoms, or are experiencing recurrent disease. A bone scan is performed only when patients complain of bone pain or skeletal metastases are suspected. Lymphangiograms are not used with children as often as they are with adults. The use of clinical staging is increasing. Pathologic staging requires a laparotomy and is performed only if the findings will change the therapy. It involves removal of the spleen and biopsies of the liver, retroperitoneal space/cavity, pelvic area, and bone marrow. Titanium cups should be placed to mark the splenic pedicle and sites of biopsies. The ovaries should be transposed to the midline position if pelvic irradiation is planned. Patients who are undergoing a splenectomy should receive *Haemophilus influenze* type B vaccine preoperatively and daily prophylactic penicillin thereafter (Hudson & Donaldson; Oberlin, 1996; Raney, 1997).

Treatment Interventions for Children or Adolescents With Hodgkin's Disease

Treatment strategies differ for the various stages of Hodgkin's disease. Patients with stage IA, IB, IIA, and IIB will, optimally, undergo a combination of chemotherapy and low-dose irradiation to the sites of disease (Yaniv et al., 1996). With stage IA, IB, and stage IIA, standard doses of radiation therapy alone could be offered to older adolescents who have completed all growth. A significant number of relapses, however, will require salvage chemotherapy. Extensive irradiation has been associated with an increased risk of developing second malignancies (e.g., breast cancer) in the radiation ports (Bhatia et al., 1996). Patients with stage IIIA and IIIB can undergo chemotherapy alone or in combination with irradiation to areas of bulky or residual disease (Schellong, 1996; Weiner et al., 1997). Patients with stage IV disease will be treated with an intensive combination protocol. Radiation therapy may be administered to areas of bulky disease (Hutchinson et al., 1998; Weiner et al.).

With recurrent Hodgkin's disease, treatment decisions will be made based on extent of disease, children's or adolescents' age, and duration of first remission (Mwanda & Othierio-Abinya, 1998). The treatment options primarily are chemotherapeutic, with bone marrow transplantation an option for patients with advanced disease.

Significant efforts have been made to reduce the amount of radiation therapy, alkylating agents, and anthracyclines included in the protocols for this disease. This will result, ideally, in reduced long-term effects and number of second malignancies for this group of survivors (Oberlin, 1996; Schellong, 1996).

Neuroblastoma

Overview

Neuroblastoma is the fourth most common childhood malignancy, with almost 550 cases diagnosed each year in the United States. It occurs more frequently among black children than among white children and is slightly more common among boys than girls, with a ratio of 1.2:1. It is the most common tumor found in children less than 1 year of age, with 36% of patients diagnosed at less than 1 year of age, 79% at less than 4 years of age, and 97% of all cases diagnosed by 10 years of age (Brodeur & Castleberry, 1997). Very rarely, fetal sonograms can detect neuroblastoma (Jennings, LaQuaglia, Leong, Hendren, & Adzick, 1993). Neuroblastoma that is diagnosed in adolescence or adulthood usually has a poor long-term prognosis, regardless of initial staging of site of disease (Franks, Bollen, Seeger, Stram, & Matthay, 1997).

Etiologic Factors Associated With Neuroblastoma

The etiology of neuroblastoma is unknown. Several studies have suggested various links between prenatal and postnatal exposures to drugs, chemicals, radiation, or electromagnetic fields, but none have been proven conclusively. Although neuroblastoma has been associated with neurofibromatosis type I and Hirschsprung disease, no other specific congenital anomalies or genetic syndromes have been reported with increased frequency with neuroblastoma (Brodeur & Castleberry, 1997). Genetic predisposition is a consideration, especially with familial neuroblastoma. In 1972, Knudson and Strong found that siblings with neuroblastoma presented at an earlier age and had multiple primary sites, suggesting an autosomal dominant pattern of inheritance (Sullivan, 1993). Kushner, Gilbert, and Helson (1986) confirmed these findings with their study of 23 siblings.

The three classic histiopathologic patterns (neuroblastoma, ganglioneuroblastoma, and ganglioneuroma) reflect a range of maturation and differentiation (Brodeur & Castleberry, 1997). Neuroblastoma consists of small, round cells with hyperchromatic nuclei and scant cytoplasm. The Homer-Wright pseudorosette, a diagnostic feature found in up to 50% of cases, is composed of neuroblasts surrounding areas of eosinophilic neuropil (Brodeur & Castleberry). Ganglioneuroblastoma tumors have areas of mature or benign cells mixed with areas of undifferentiated or malignant cells (Sullivan, 1993). These tumors may be focal or diffuse, but diffuse ganglioneuroblastoma is associated with less aggressive behavior (Brodeur & Castleberry). Ganglioneuroma is a benign, fully differentiated tumor that is composed principally of mature ganglion cells, neuropil, and Schwann cells (Brodeur & Castleberry). These histiopathologic differences may be present within the tumor or between the primary site and the metastatic areas of disease (Azizkhan & Haase, 1993; Brodeur & Castleberry; Sullivan).

Several biological variables are present in children with neuroblastoma that may affect treatment decisions. Amplification of the N-myc oncogene, present in cell lines of neuroblastoma, correlated highly with rapid tumor progression and overall poor prognosis (Tonini et al., 1997). Expression of other oncogenes, such as HRAS, correlates with lower disease stages (Brodeur & Castleberry, 1997). DNA analysis by flow cytometry is a simple test that correlates with biologic behaviors. Hyperdiploidy DNA content in infants (DI > 1) correlates with lower stages of disease and a better response to chemotherapeutic agents. In older patients, however, this does not correlate with a favorable outcome. Cytogenetically, the deletion of the short arm of chromosome 1, which is thought to represent the loss of the neuroblastoma suppressor gene, characterizes neuroblastomas. Some studies have found the human multidrug resistance gene (MDR1) in some neuroblastoma cells. High levels of p-glycoprotein, the protein product of MDR1, corresponds with the development of resistance to chemotherapy and a poor prognosis (Sullivan, 1993). Elevation of the urinary excreted VMA or HVA, elevated serum ferritin, serum neuron-specific enolase (NSE), and LDH correlate with poor prognosis (Brodeur & Castleberry). The Shimada classification system involves clinical and histologic parameters such as age, stage, and tumor morphology to determine prognosis (Joshi et al., 1992).

Three major staging systems are used for neuroblastoma: CCG staging system, POG staging system (also used by St. Jude Children's Research Hospital), and the International Neuroblastoma Staging System (INSS). Table 3-9 summarizes a comparison of these three systems. INSS has features of both the CCG and POG systems and currently is being analyzed by both groups. Current treatment protocols employ either the CCG or POG staging guidelines to determine treatment while also assigning an INSS stage. The goal is to validate the staging process of INSS so that, in the future, only one staging system will be accepted worldwide (Castleberry et al., 1994).

Clinical Presentation of Neuroblastoma in Children

The initial symptoms that are associated with neuroblastoma are related to the area of disease. Sixty-five percent of primary tumors develop in the abdomen. Forty percent of these develop in the adrenal glands. Twenty-five percent develop in the paraspinal ganglia. A primary tumor cannot be found in approximately 1% of patients (Brodeur & Castleberry, 1997). Less common primary sites are the paraspinal area of the thorax (15%), neck (5%), and pelvis (5%) (Sullivan, 1993). Patients can present with more than one primary site of disease. Disseminated disease is found in 68% of older children at diagnosis. Neuroblastoma can metastasize to regional lymph nodes, lymph nodes beyond the original site, bone marrow, bone, liver, skin, and, very rarely, to the lungs or brain (Azizkhan & Haase, 1993; Brodeur & Castleberry).

Children who present with abdominal disease have progressing complaints of pain, fullness, and occasional gastrointestinal disease symptoms (e.g., bleeding, bowel obstruction). A hard, irregular abdominal mass can be palpated during examination. Retroperitoneal abdominal and pelvic tumors that are large can cause compression of venous and lymphatic drainage from the lower extremities and lead to scrotal and lower extremity edema (Brodeur & Castleberry, 1997). A chest x-ray can detect masses in the thorax. If large enough, the masses can cause respiratory symptoms or

Table 3-9. Comparison of Staging Systems for Neuroblastoma

Children's Cancer Study Group (CCSG) System	Pediatric Oncology Group (POG) System	International Neuroblastoma Staging System (INSS)
Stage I Tumor confined to the organ or structure of origin	**Stage A** Complete gross resection of primary tumor, with or without microscopic residual disease; intracavitary lymph nodes not adhered to primary tumor and histologically free of tumor; nodes adhered to the surface of or within primary tumor possibly positive	**Stage 1** Localized tumor confined to the area of origin; complete gross excision, with or without microscopic residual disease; identifiable ipsilateral and contralateral lymph nodes negative microscopically
Stage II Tumor extending in continuity beyond the organ or structure of origin but not crossing the midline; regional lymph nodes on the ipsilateral side possibly involved	**Stage B** Grossly unresected primary tumor; nodes and nodules the same as in stage A	**Stage 2A** Unilateral tumor with incomplete gross excision; identifiable ipsilateral and contralateral lymph nodes negative microscopically **Stage 2B** Unilateral tumor with complete or incomplete gross excision; with positive ipsilateral regional lymph nodes; identifiable contralateral lymph nodes negative microscopically
Stage III Tumor extending in continuity beyond the midline; regional lymph nodes possibly involved bilaterally	**Stage C** Complete or incomplete resection of primary tumor; intracavitary nodes not adhered to primary tumor histologically positive for tumor; liver as in stage A	**Stage 3** Tumor infiltrating across the midline with or without regional lymph node involvement; or unilateral tumor with contralateral regional lymph node involvement; or midline tumor with bilateral lymph node involvement
Stage IV Remote disease involving the skeleton, bone marrow, soft tissue, and distant lymph node groups (see stage IV-S)	**Stage D** Dissemination of disease beyond intracavitary nodes (e.g., extracavitary nodes, liver, skin, bone marrow, bone)	**Stage 4** Dissemination of tumor to distant lymph nodes, bone, bone marrow, liver, or other organs (except as defined as stage 4S)
Stage IV-S As defined in stage I or II, except for the presence of remote disease confined to the liver, skin, or marrow (without bone metastases)	**Stage DS** Infants < one year of age with stage IV-S disease (see CCSF)	**Stage 4S** Localized primary tumor as defined for stage 1 or 2 with dissemination limited to liver, skin, or bone marrow

Note. From "Neuroblastoma" (p. 777) by G.M. Brodeur and R.P. Castleberry in P.A. Pizzo and D.G. Poplack (Eds.) *Principles and Practice of Pediatric Oncology* (3rd ed.), 1997, Philadelphia: Lippincott-Raven Publishers. Copyright 1997 by Lippincott-Raven Publishers. Reprinted with permission.

superior vena cava syndrome from mechanical obstruction. A high thoracic or cervical tumor can cause Horner's syndrome, which is a result of paralysis of the cervical sympathetic nerve trunk. Paraspinal tumors can extend into the neural foramina of the vertebral bodies and produce symptoms caused by compression of nerve roots and spinal cord (Brodeur & Castleberry; Sullivan, 1993).

Metastatic neuroblastoma can present in many ways. Ecchymosis of the eyelids and proptosis result from retrobulbar and orbital infiltration by tumor. Bone and bone marrow disease (Hutchinson syndrome) usually present as pain that causes limping and, in some cases, inability to walk. If the bone marrow is replaced with tumor, signs of bone marrow failure (e.g., anemia, thrombocytopenia) may be present. Progression of generalized symptoms (e.g., failure to thrive, irritability, fever associated with bone metastases) may become exacerbated.

Unique paraneoplastic syndromes are associated with neuroblastoma. The opsoclonus/myoclonus syndrome, characterized by random eye movements and myoclonic jerking, is believed to have an immunologic mechanism and usually is associated with low-grade disease. The survival rate is good, but, despite treatment with chemotherapy, steroids, gammaglobulin, or adrenocorticotropic hormone, children are often left with severe, permanent neurologic disabilities (e.g., psychomotor retardation) (Russo, Cohn, Petruzzi, & deAlarcon, 1997). Tumor secretion of vasoactive intestinal peptide causes intractable diarrhea leading to hypokalemia and dehydration (Kerner-Morrison syndrome). Removal of the tumor usually resolves the symptoms, and these patients have a good outcome (Azizkhan & Haase, 1993; Brodeur & Castleberry, 1997).

Diagnostic Evaluation of Children With Neuroblastoma

When children present with suspected neuroblastoma, obtaining a detailed health history and performing a thorough physical examination are important. The initial laboratory work should include a complete blood count, liver and kidney function tests, a coagulation profile, and measurements of tumor markers such as catecholamine metabolites (VMA and HVA), ferritin, NSE, and ganglioside GD_2. Measuring the VMA and HVA in urine is reliable (Brodeur & Castleberry, 1997; Franks et al., 1997).

The following are the minimum recommended investigations for determining extent of disease. Bone marrow samples should be analyzed from bilateral posterior iliac crest marrow aspirates and core bone marrow biopsies. An iodine 131-metaiodobenzylguanadine scan (MIBG) to evaluate bone and soft tissue disease should be performed. A bone scan should be performed if the MIBG is unavailable or is negative. Palpable lymph nodes should be examined clinically and histologically. CT or MRI should be performed to evaluate liver, spleen, and nonpalpable lymph nodes using three-dimensional measurements. A chest x-ray using anterior and posterior images is performed initially and followed by CT or MRI if disease is detected (Brodeur et al., 1993; Castleberry et al., 1994).

Treatment Interventions for Children With Neuroblastoma

Treatment for neuroblastoma is based on multiple factors such as stage, patients' age, the Shimada grade, ferritin, NSE, LDH, N-myc amplification, and DNA ploidy. The specific therapeutic protocol is decided for each patient after the complete workup is evaluated (Brodeur et al., 1993; Joshi et al., 1992; Tonini et al., 1997).

Patients with localized disease have a cure rate greater than 90%. These include INSS stage I, CCG stage II or III tumors that have been resected and have negative nodes, POG stage A and favorable biologic features. Cure is achieved usually through gross total surgical resection alone (Kushner et al., 1996). Long-term survival for patients with localized, unresectable disease is 75%–90%, which includes patients with INSS stage II, CCG stage I, II, or III tumors that are not resected completely and have negative nodes, and POG stage B disease. These patients, depending on all other prognostic features, undergo initial surgery followed by chemotherapy. If disease is present at the second-look surgery, radiation may be administered. The length of therapy is usually four to six months (Garaventa et al., 1993; Matthay et al., 1998). Patients with INSS stage III, CCG stage II or III with positive nodes, and POG stage III disease have treatment options and overall survival rates that differ with age. Infants younger than one year have ≥ 80% chance of cure. Complete surgical resection, either at diagnosis or after the tumor has responded to therapy, can improve survival (Azizkhan & Haase, 1993). The chemotherapeutic agents used are cyclophosphamide, doxorubicin, cisplatin, teniposide, or etoposide (Brodeur & Castleberry, 1997). Children who are older than one year have a somewhat lower cure rate despite the use of more aggressive therapy. Complete resection of the tumor should be a goal either initially or after a treatment response. Intensive combinations of the same drugs will be used with the younger children (Bowman et al., 1997). Localized radiation therapy also may be used. Children older than one year with a more dismal prognosis as determined by the presence of prognostic indicators will undergo a more intensive plan of therapy involving high-dose chemotherapy and radiation therapy followed by bone marrow transplantation (Saarinen et al., 1996).

Stage IV-S (in the CCG staging system), stage DS (in the POG staging system), or stage 4S (in the INSS) is a "special" neuroblastoma that usually develops in infants less than one year of age and can spontaneously regress. Therapy generally is not needed, although these children need to be monitored carefully throughout time (Guglielmi et al., 1996). Children with disseminated disease at diagnosis are those in CCG stage IV, POG stage D, or INSS stage IV. Children who are younger than one year have somewhat better outcomes than older children. Intensive therapy may include chemotherapy, radiation therapy, surgery, autologous or allogeneic bone marrow transplant, bone marrow rescue, and immunotherapy with monoclonal antibodies that are specific to neuroblastoma (e.g., 3F8) (Kushner et al., 1994; Sullivan, 1993). The advent of cytokines (e.g., G-CSF) has made treating patients more aggressively in a shorter time span possible. After a series of pilot studies, CCG concluded that progression-free survival of patients with high-risk neuroblastoma was improved with the use of autologous purged bone marrow transplantation or allogeneic transplantation. Recurrent or progressive neuroblastoma is treated according to the extent of disease. It is usually widespread and carries a poor prognosis despite aggressive therapy. The combination of autologous stem cell transplantation and 13-cis retinoic acid has shown promise in treating those with high-risk neuroblastoma (Khan, Villablanca, Reynolds, & Avramis, 1996).

Future research regarding neuroblastoma should focus on identifying individuals with a genetic predisposition to the disease through effective screening, identifying additional tumor markers, further identifying prognostic indicators, and developing biologically directed therapy with less toxicities than current treatment protocols (Brodeur & Castleberry, 1997). Screening for neuroblastoma currently is being evaluated, although it is not believed to decrease overall mortality and morbidity (Woods et al., 1996).

Bone Tumors

Overview

Malignant bone tumors account for approximately 6% of all childhood malignancies. The major bone tumors are osteosarcomas, which make up about 60% of the cases, and Ewing's sarcoma, which comprises about 30% of all cases. Several other tumors make up the remaining 10% of bone tumors.

Osteosarcoma

Overview

Osteosarcoma is the most common primary malignant bone tumor in children and adolescents. The peak incidence occurs between 10 and 22 years of age, with a higher incidence found in adolescent and young adult males. It is the third most common cancer in adolescents. Approximately 900 cases of osteosarcoma of the bone are diagnosed in children, adolescents, and young adults each year in the United States.

Much needs to be learned about the causes of osteosarcoma. A correlation seems to exist between rapid bone growth and the development of this tumor because the peak incidence age corresponds with the adolescent growth spurt. Osteosarcoma, however, also develops in patients before and after the adolescent growth spurt (Meyers & Gorlick, 1997). Exposure to radiation is a known cause of osteosarcoma. A genetic predisposition to this tumor may exist. Reports of families in which more than one case of osteosarcoma was diagnosed exist. Patients with hereditary retinoblastoma have an increased risk for developing osteosarcoma. Data confirm that the specific locus involved in the generation of retinoblastoma also is implicated in the generation of osteosarcoma, even in patients without retinoblastoma (Link & Eilber, 1997).

Osteosarcoma can present in any bone in the body. The most common primary sites are the long bones, with the distal femur being the most frequent primary site followed by the proximal tibia and proximal humerus. Approximately 10%–20% of patients will present with metastatic disease, although a much higher percentage of patients are believed to have subclinical microscopic metastasis at presentation (Meyers & Gorlick, 1997). The lungs are the most common area for metastatic disease, although it can spread to other bones, kidneys, pleura, adrenal glands, brain, and the pericardium (Link & Eilber, 1997).

Clinical Presentation and Evaluation of Children and Adolescents With Osteosarcoma

The presenting symptoms of patients with osteosarcoma are pain at the affected area or referred pain to areas such as the hip or back. Symptoms usually are present for several months and are attributed initially to trauma or increased physical exercise, which causes the delay in diagnosis. On examination, local edema, enlargement of a localized area, pain on palpation, decreased range of motion, redness, and, occasionally, a pulsation or bruit may exist (Betcher, 1993).

The evaluation of children with suspected osteosarcoma begins with a detailed history followed by a physical examination. Radiographic studies include plain films of the primary site followed by a CT or MRI using cross-sectional imaging techniques. This will help to define the extent of tumor within the bone, extent of soft tissue mass, any involvement of adjacent joint space, and relationships with vital structures such as blood vessels and nerves (Meyers & Gorlick, 1997). A radionuclide bone scan will help to further define the extent of the primary tumor and identify skip and metastatic lesions. A skip lesion is a separate lesion present in the same bone as the original tumor, while a metastatic lesion is present in a distant site. A chest CT will identify possible lung metastasis. Serum evaluations should include a complete blood count and chemistry profile, including alkaline phosphatase and LDH. Systemic chemotherapy must be used to successfully treat this disease. The following baseline evaluations must be made prior to beginning therapy: a creatinine clearance to evaluate renal function, an audiogram to evaluate hearing, and an echocardiogram to evaluate cardiac function. In addition, postpubertal males should be encouraged to bank their sperm because sterility is a side effect of many of the chemotherapeutic agents used.

Pathologic examination of the tumor tissue through a biopsy definitively diagnoses osteosarcoma. Meyers and Gorlick (1997) strongly suggest the use of an open biopsy because it allows an experienced surgeon to obtain the tissue necessary for complete pathologic and biologic studies while leaving all future surgical therapeutic options open for an orthopedic oncologist.

Histologically, osteosarcomas develop from primitive mesenchymal cells and are usually malignant osteoblasts and spindle cells that form an extracellular matrix of osteoid. WHO's histologic classification of bone tumors separates the osteosarcomas into central (medullary) and surface (peripheral) tumors, with a number of subtypes within each group (Schajowicz, Sissons, & Sobbin, 1995). The most common pathologic subtype is the conventional central osteosarcoma, which is characterized by areas of necrosis, atypical mitosis, and malignant cartilage and found predominantly in children and adolescents. Grading osteosarcomas is difficult, although the majority are judged to be high-grade (Link & Eilber, 1997). Localized disease means that the tumor is limited to the original bone. The presence of local skip lesions at diagnosis may or may not affect the overall prognosis, and it remains an area of controversy. Metastatic disease indicates visible spread to other areas at diagnosis and is present in 10%–20% of patients. It indicates a worse prognosis.

Treatment Interventions for Children and Adolescents With Osteosarcoma

Successful treatment of osteosarcoma requires systemic chemotherapy (Meyers & Gorlick, 1997). The most commonly used chemotherapeutic agents are doxorubicin, cisplatin, high-dose methotrexate with leucovorin rescue, cyclophosphamide, and ifosfamide. For patients with localized disease, preoperative or induction chemotherapy is administered in an attempt to increase the likelihood of performing a limb-sparing surgical procedure and to decrease the chance of metastatic spread of the disease. After the administration of the initial chemotherapy, the surgical procedure is performed (either amputation or limb salvage). Adjuvant postoperative chemotherapy then is administered (Provisor et al., 1997). High-dose localized irradiation may be added to the treatment regimen for localized but inoperable lesions. For patients with metastatic disease, very aggressive multiagent chemotherapy in conjunction with surgery and, possibly, radiation therapy are necessary. The primary and metastatic disease should be removed surgically when possible. Even when all detectable disease has been removed, aggressive high-dose chemotherapy should be administered (Meyers et al., 1993).

Patients with recurrent or progressive metastatic disease to the lungs may be eligible only for surgical resection. At first relapse, the ability to completely resect pulmonary tumors enhances the survival rate (Tabone et al., 1994). The overall prognosis is poor for patients who have recurrent or progressive disease that is inoperable. The treatment plan used at the time of recurrence depends on many factors, including location of disease, prior therapy, and degree of surgical accessibility. Ifosfamide has been shown to be effective against recurrent osteosarcoma in a POG study (Harris et al., 1995).

Prognostic Indicators

Many factors affect prognosis. In general, the use of adjuvant chemotherapy greatly improves outcome. With localized disease, treatment of distal tumors has a more favorable outcome. Resectability is important because these tumors do not respond to radiation therapy. Higher levels of serum LDH or alkaline phosphatase predict a poorer outcome (Meyers & Gorlick, 1997). Patients with more than 95% necrosis in the primary tumor have a better prognosis than those with less tumor necrosis (Davis, Bell, & Goodwin 1994). Overall, patients who present with metastatic disease have a dismal survival rate.

Future Considerations

During the last 25 years, dramatic strides have been made in improving the overall survival rates of osteosarcoma. This is a result of many factors, including the use of adjuvant chemotherapy, significant advances in diagnostic imaging, the use of innovative orthopedic oncology procedures, and improved rehabilitation services. Ongoing studies, such as those being performed by POG and CCG to evaluate the use of ifosfamide in treating recurrent disease and muramyl tripeptide phosphatidylethanolamine to prevent metastatic disease, ideally will continue to improve the disease-free survival rates of all patients with osteosarcoma (Meyers & Gorlick, 1997).

Ewing's Family of Tumors

Overview

The Ewing's family of tumors (EFTs) includes Ewing's tumors or Ewing's sarcoma of bone, extraosseus Ewing's, primitive neuroectodermal tumors (peripheral neuroepithelioma), and Askin's tumors (peripheral neuroepithelioma of the chest wall). This family of tumors is a spectrum of a single biologic entity (Horowitz, Malawer, Woo, & Hicks, 1997).

The peak incidence of EFTs is between ages 10 and 20. They are slightly more common among males than females, with a ratio of 1.1:1, and are rarely diagnosed among nonwhites. Ewing's tumors of bone comprise approximately 60% of the EFTs and develop most commonly in the extremities, pelvis, chest, spine, and skull. Extraosseus Ewing's develops most commonly in the trunk, retroperitoneum, extremities, and head and neck. Common sites of the peripheral neuroepithelioma include the chest, abdomen, pelvis, extremities, and head and neck (Raney et al., 1997).

The etiology of this disease entity is unknown. No strong congenital or hereditary correlations exist. Reports of such associations are rare. These tumors rarely occur as secondary malignant neoplasms.

Clinical Presentation and Evaluation of Children and Adolescents With a Ewing's Family Tumor

The presenting symptoms of patients who are suspected of having this disease depend on the site of disease and the amount of disease present at diagnosis. Patients can experience symptoms for months before the diagnosis is confirmed. Pain is the most common symptom. On examination, a mass may or may not be palpable. Pathologic fractures can occur and are caused by tumor invasion of the bone. A history of unexplained fevers is fairly common.

The evaluation of children or adolescents begins with a detailed history and physical examination. Radiographic studies will begin with plain films of the primary site. A CT scan is performed to aid in defining the extent of disease. An MRI can provide information about the presence of marrow and soft tissue disease and the relationship between the tumor and surrounding blood vessels and nerves. A bone scan and gallium scan will help to further define the bony extent of the tumor and aid in detecting metastatic areas of disease. A bone marrow aspirate and biopsy must be performed in one or more sites. Baseline serum laboratory work should include a complete blood count and chemistry profile, including hepatic and renal evaluations. An elevated serum LDH level is a poor prognostic indicator. Prior to beginning systemic therapy, children or adolescents must have baseline renal, audiology, cardiology, and pulmonary testing performed. Postpubertal males should be encouraged to bank their sperm.

The biopsy provides the definitive diagnosis. When possible, the tissue specimen should be taken from the extraosseous component rather than from the bone to prevent fractures following radiation therapy (Horowitz et al., 1997). A skilled oncology surgeon who will be involved in future surgical interventions should perform a biopsy.

Histologically, EFTs range from typical, undifferentiated Ewing's sarcoma to atypical, poorly differentiated Ewing's sarcoma to differentiated peripheral neuroepithelioma (Horowitz et al., 1997). They are malignant tumors that are histologically characterized by uniform, tightly packed, small, round cells with oval to round nuclei and indistinct cytoplasm, and they are without nucleoli (Delattre et al., 1994). Despite some differentiation between the tumors, the significant overlap of many histopathologic features supports the theory that this group of neoplasms is a single entity. This range of tumors shares the same genetic features, including a t(11,22) translocation.

Staging of the disease refers to the amount of disease at diagnosis. Localized disease is defined as disease that has not, by clinical and imaging techniques, spread beyond the original site or regional lymph nodes. In actuality, however, a high percentage of patients (approximately 90%) have occult metastatic disease at diagnosis. Extraosseus Ewing's has been grouped according to the following rhabdomyosarcoma staging system: Group I (completely excised), Group II (microscopic residual), and Group III (gross residual) (Raney et al., 1997). Metastatic tumors are those that have spread to distant sites. The most common areas of metastases are lung, bone, and bone marrow.

Treatment Interventions for Children and Adolescents With a Ewing's Family Tumor

A multimodality approach to EFTs includes multidrug chemotherapy, radiation therapy, or surgical therapy (Madero et al., 1998). The most commonly used chemotherapeutic agents include vincristine, doxorubicin, and cyclophosphamide and are alternated with ifosfamide and etoposide. Patients who appear to have localized disease at diagnosis are treated with multidrug chemotherapy, surgery, or irradiation as needed. Surgery is the preferred option if resection of the tumor is possible (Scully et al., 1995). Radiation therapy is reserved for patients who do not have a surgical option or cases of incomplete resection or a resection with inadequate margins. Radiation therapy involves precise treatment planning to accomplish control of the tumor while preserving surrounding healthy tissue (Donaldson et al., 1998). In some cases, surgery becomes an option after shrinkage of the tumor with radiation therapy.

Patients with metastatic disease have an overall poor prognosis. Treatment includes intensive chemotherapy combined with radiation therapy to each site of disease. Surgical excision of tumor sites is performed when possible (Kushner et al., 1995). Protocols incorporating high-dose chemotherapy with peripheral stem cell rescue are used to treat patients with extensive disease. Total body irradiation also may be used (Burdach et al., 1993). Patients who have only lung metastases have a slightly better prognosis than those with metastases to bone, bone marrow, or other areas.

Patients presenting with recurrent disease after completion of therapy have a somewhat better prognosis than those whose disease progresses while undergoing therapy. Overall, the prognosis is poor. The treatment plan used depends on factors such as amount of disease, prior treatment, and issues particular to the individual child or adolescent. Aggressive multimodal treatment protocols are used to control further disease spread while treating the clinically obvious areas (Burdach et al., 1993).

The most important prognostic indicator of EFTs is the absence of clinical metastatic disease at diagnosis. Primary site of disease is indicative of outcome, with distal bones and ribs being the most favorable site. Initial tumor size can affect prognosis. Tumors larger than 100 cubic centimeters have a less favorable disease-free survival rate. An initial good response to treatment and younger age at diagnosis are good indicators. Patients with initial normal serum LDH levels had significantly better outcomes than those with high levels (Horowitz et al., 1997).

Current research is aimed at intensifying therapy for high-risk patients while using bone marrow and peripheral blood stem cell support. Increased understanding of the molecular mechanisms that cause EFTs ideally will result in more sophisticated methods of detecting disease, new drugs aimed directly at the specific genetic component of these tumors, and more intense combination protocols using bone marrow and peripheral blood stem cell rescues with high-risk patients (Horowitz et al., 1997; Madero et al., 1998).

Long-Term Effects for Pediatric Cancer Survivors

With the success of aggressive treatment of many childhood cancers, more children and adolescents are experiencing long-term survival (see Table 3-1). The more aggressive multimodality treatment protocols bring with them a set of long-term problems that need to be monitored and addressed systematically. A wide range of areas (e.g., physical, psychological, educational, behavioral) may be affected. The adverse effects encountered by survivors depend on age at diagnosis, disease entity, specific treatment protocol, and follow-up support given after treatment is completed. Early intervention may lessen the degree of problems encountered by individuals.

The physical effects are specific to each organ system and may require specialized monitoring and intervention. Either direct damage to organs (e.g., damage to the testes, ovaries, or thyroid) or the controlling hypothalamic pituitary axis can result in dysfunction of the endocrine system (Hobbie, Ruccione, Moore, & Truesdell, 1993; Sklar, 1997). Difficulties with the central nervous system can manifest themselves as other neuropsychologic deficits as well as actual physical anatomic abnormalities (e.g., white matter atrophy) (Copeland, Moore, Francis, Jaffe, & Culbert, 1996; Sklar, 1997). Cardiovascular problems may present acutely or develop throughout time. The effects usually are apparent and long-term and result from cumulative treatment dose. Damage to the respiratory system can present as acute pneumonitis or chronic fibrosis. Management will depend on the severity of the specific entity. Growth impairment and development reflect late effects to the musculoskeletal system (Sklar, 1995). Problems with the condition of the teeth, salivary glands, and the oral cavity in general are concerns. The kidneys and bladder can exhibit problems if the urinary tract has been affected. The gastrointestinal tract can be affected from the esophagus down to the rectum, resulting in a wide range of symptoms. Varying degrees of pancytopenia as well as immunosuppression indicate damage to the hematopoietic system. Mild to severe late effects on vision and hearing can greatly affect daily functioning. Underlying disease, prior treatment, and the cytoreductive regimen used for transplantation or the development of chronic graft versus host disease can compound the late effects that result from bone marrow transplantation (Boulad, Sands, & Sklar, 1998). The most devastating consequence of childhood cancer therapy is the development of second malignancies (Marina, 1997). Leukemia and solid tumors are the most common of these malignancies. Survivors also can exhibit difficulties in psychological, educational, social, and behavioral arenas. The younger children are when they are diagnosed, the higher their risk for developing cognitive and behavioral late effects (Eiser, 1998). Early intervention has been shown to have significant positive outcomes with psychological late effects.

Educating pediatric cancer survivors in regard to their physical and mental health risks is imperative and will encourage them to comply with follow-up monitoring, which should occur throughout their lifetime. Specialists in long-term effects should care for these individuals so that concerns will be monitored and interventions will be rapid. Multidisciplinary teams specializing in the long-term effects of pediatric cancer should care for survivors and address all facets of concern. In addition to providing physical care during each visit, anticipatory guidance and education should be given about possible late effects, appropriate development, and psychological and social issues. Support groups for survivors can address specific issues while creating a forum in which individuals can discuss their personal struggles.

Many institutions are conducting formalized studies focusing on the physical and psychological well-being of survivors. The National Cancer Institute (NCI) Office of Cancer Survivorship began to organize important areas of research on survivorship in 1996. In late 1998, NCI awarded $15 million over five years for new studies of cancer survivors.

Survivors of childhood cancer are a growing population with unique concerns. To ensure a continually high quality of life, each of these concerns must be recognized and addressed adequately. In addition, continued surveillance of this population is essential to monitor the impact of the therapeutic modifications on late complications and potentially to detect the sequelae produced by newer treatment strategies (Marina, 1997). Ideally, this will assist pediatric oncologists in developing future treatment strategies that will minimize additional long-term effects.

Conclusion

All professionals involved with the care of children or adolescents with cancer are working toward achieving a cure while preserving the highest quality of life possible. These children must be treated in pediatric cancer centers by meticulous multidisciplinary teams who are knowledgeable about all facets of childhood cancer. Continuing to heighten public awareness of childhood cancer is important so that necessary research programs will be funded adequately. Despite the overall positive trend in survival rates, some cancers remain resistant to treatment. The ultimate goal is to achieve a cure for each of the childhood cancers that are diagnosed each day. Researchers will continue to strive to determine the causes of cancer in children so that effective preventive measures can be formulated and implemented.

References

Anderson, J.R., Jenkin, R.D., Wilson, J.K, Kieldsberg, C., Sposto, R., Chilcote, R., Coccia, P., Exelby, P., Siegel, S., Meadows, A.T., & Hammond, G.D. (1993). Long term follow-up of patients treated with COMP or LSA2L2 therapy for childhood non-Hodgkin's lymphoma: A report of CCG-551 from the Children's Cancer Group. *Journal of Clinical Oncology, 11,* 1024–1032.

Ater, J. (1998). Treatment of brain tumors in children: An overview. *Journal of Care Management, 4,* 96–108.

Azizkhan, R.G., & Haase, G.M. (1993). Current biologic and therapeutic implications in the surgery of neuroblastoma. *Seminars in Surgical Oncology, 9,* 493–501.

Balis, F.M., Hokenberg, J.S., & Poplack, D.G. (1997). General principles of chemotherapy. In P.A. Pizzo & D.G. Poplack (Eds.), *Principles and practice of pediatric oncology* (3rd ed.) (pp. 215–272). Philadelphia: Lippincott-Raven.

Beral, V., & Newton, R. (1998). Overview of the epidemiology of immunodeficiency-associated cancers. *Journal of the National Cancer Institute Monographs, 23,* 1–6.

Bergeron, S. (1998). A review of the past, present, and future clinical trials from the Children's Cancer Group. *Journal of Pediatric Oncology Nursing, 15,* 98–102.

Betcher, D. (1993). Bone tumors. In G.V. Foley, G. Fochtman, & K.H. Mooney (Eds.), *Nursing care of the child with cancer* (2nd ed.) (pp. 300–309). Philadelphia: W.B. Saunders.

Bhatia, S., Robison, L.L., Oberlin, O., Greenberg, M., Bunim, G., Fossati-Bellani, F., & Meadows, A.T. (1996). Breast cancer and other second neoplasms after childhood Hodgkin's disease. *New England Journal of Medicine, 334,* 745–751.

Bouffet, E., Perilongo, G., Canete, A., & Massimimo, M. (1998). Intracranial ependymomas in children: A critical review of prognostic factors and a plea for cooperation. *Medical and Pediatric Oncology, 30,* 319–329.

Boulad, F., Sands, S., & Sklar, C. (1998). Late complications after bone marrow transplantation in children and adolescents. *Current Problems in Pediatrics, 28*(9), 277–297.

Bowman, L.C., Castleberry, R.P., Cantor, A., Joshi, V., Cohn, S.L., Smith, E.J., Yu, A., Brodeur, G.M., Hayes, F.A., & Look, A.T. (1997). Genetic staging of unresectable or metastatic neuroblastoma in infants: A Pediatric Oncology Group study. *Journal of the National Cancer Institute, 89,* 373–380.

Bowman, W.P., Shuster, J.J., Cook, B., Griffin, T., Behm, F., Pullen, J., Link, M., Head, D., Carroll, A., Berard, C., & Murphy, S. (1996). Improved survival for children with b-cell acute lymphoblastic leukemia and stage IV small non-cleaved cell lymphoma: A pediatric oncology group study. *Journal of Clinical Oncology, 14,* 1252–1261.

Brodeur, G.M., & Castleberry, R.P. (1997). Neuroblastoma. In P.A. Pizzo & D.G. Poplack (Eds.), *Principles and practice of pediatric oncology* (3rd ed.) (pp. 761–797). Philadelphia: Lippincott-Raven.

Brodeur, G.M., Pritchard, J., Berthhold, F., Carlsen, N.L., Caste, I.V., Castleberry, R.P., Bernardi, B.D., Evans, A.E., Favrot, M., Hedborg, F., Kaneko, M., Kemshead, J., Fritz, L., Lee, R.E., Look, A.T., Pearson, A.D., Philip, T., Roald, B., Sawade, T., Seeger, R.C., Tsuchida, Y., & Voute, P.A. (1993). Revisions of the international criteria for neuroblastoma diagnosis, staging, and response to treatment. *Journal of Clinical Oncology, 11,* 1466–1477.

Burdach, S., Jurgens, H., Peters, C., Nurnberger, W., Mauz-Korholz, C., Korholz, D., Paulussen, M., Pape, H., Dilloo, D., Koscielniak, E., Gadner, H., & Gobal, U. (1993). Myeloablative radiochemotherapy and hematopoietic stem cell rescue in poor prognosis Ewing's sarcoma. *Journal of Clinical Oncology, 11,* 1482–1488.

Castleberry, R.P., Shuster, J.J., Smith, E.I., & Member Institutions of the Pediatric Oncology Group. (1994). The Pediatric Oncology Group experience with the International Staging System criteria for neuroblastoma. *Journal of Clinical Oncology, 12,* 2378–2381.

Cohen, M.E., & Duffman, P. (Eds.). (1994). *Brain tumors in children: Principles of diagnosis and treatment* (2nd ed.). New York: Raven Press.

Copeland, D.R., Moore, B.D., III, Francis, D.J., Jaffe, N., & Culbert, S.J. (1996). Neuropsychologic effects of chemotherapy on children with cancer: A longitudinal study. *Journal of Clinical Oncology, 14,* 2826–2835.

Davis, A.M., Bell, R.S., & Goodwin, R.J. (1994). Prognostic factors in osteosarcoma: A critical review. *Journal of Clinical Oncology, 12,* 423–431.

Delattre, O., Zucman, J., Melot, T., Garau, S., Zucker, J.M., Lenoir, G.M., Ambros, P.F., Sheer, D., Turc-Caral, C., Triche, T.J., Aurias, A., & Thomas, G. (1994). The Ewing family of tumors—A subgroup of small round cell tumors defined by specific chimeric transcripts. *New England Journal of Medicine, 331,* 294–299.

Deutsch, M., Thomas, P.R., Krischer, J., Boyett, J.M., Albright, L., Aronin, P., Langston, J., Allen, J.C., Packer, R.J., Linggood, R., Mulberm, R., Stanley, P., Stenbens, J.A., Duffner, P., Kun, L., Rorke, L., Cherlow, J., Friedman, H., Finlay, J.L., & Vietti, T. (1996). Results of a prospective randomized trial comparing standard dose neuraxis irradiation (3600 cGy/20) with reduced neuraxis irradiation (2340 cGy/13) in patients with low-stage and medulloblastoma: A combined Children's Cancer Group-Pediatric Oncology Group study. *Pediatric Neurosurgery, 24*(4), 167–177.

Donaldson, S.S., Torrey, M., Link, M.P., Glicksman, A., Gilula, L., Laurie, F., Manning, J., Neff, J., Reinus, W., Thompson, E., & Shuster, J.J. (1998). A multidisciplinary study investigating radiotherapy in Ewing's sarcoma: End results of POG #8346. *International Journal of Radiation Oncology, Biology, Physics, 42,* 125–135.

Duffner, P.K., Horowitz, M.E., Krischer, J.P., Friedman, H.S., Burger, P.C., Cohen, M.E., Sanford, R.A., Mulhern, R.K., James, H.E., & Freeman, C.R. (1993). Postoperative chemotherapy and delayed radiation in children less than three years of age with malignant brain tumors. *New England Journal of Medicine, 328,* 1725–1731.

Dunkel, I.J., Boyett, J.M., Yates, A., Rosenblum, M., Garvin, J.H., Bostrom, B.C., Goldman, S., Sender, L.S., Gardner, S.L., Hao, L., Allen, J.C., & Finlay, J.L. (1998). For the Children's Cancer Group: High-dose carboplatin, thiotepa, and etoposide with autologous stem cell rescue for patients with recurrent medulloblastoma. *Journal of Clinical Oncology, 16,* 222–228.

Dunkel, I.J., & Finlay, J.L. (1996). High-dose chemotherapy with autologous stem cell rescue for patients with medulloblastoma. *Journal of Neuro-Oncology, 29,* 69–74.

Ebb, D.H., & Weinstein, H.J. (1997). Diagnosis and treatment of childhood acute myelogenous leukemia. *Pediatric Clinics of North America, 44,* 847–862.

Eiser, C. (1998). Practitioner review: Long-term consequences of childhood cancer. *Journal of Clinical Psychology and Psychiatry and Allied Disciplines, 39,* 621–633.

Evans, W.E., Relling, M.V., Rodman, J.H., Crom, W.R., Boyett, J.M., & Pui, C.H. (1998). Conventional compared with individualized chemotherapy for childhood acute lymphoblastic leukemia. *New England Journal of Medicine, 338,* 499–505.

Foley, G.V., & Fergusson, J.M. (1993). History, issues and trends. In G.V. Foley, G. Fochtman, & K.H. Mooney (Eds.), *Nursing care of the child with cancer* (2nd ed.) (pp. 1–24). Philadelphia: W.B. Saunders.

Franks, L.M., Bollen, A., Seeger, R.C., Stram, D.O., & Matthay, K.K. (1997). Neuroblastoma in adults and adolescents: An indolent course with poor survival. *Cancer, 79,* 2028–2035.

Freeman, C.R., & Farmer, J.P. (1998). Pediatric brain stem gliomas: A review. *International Journal of Radiation Oncology, Biology, Physics, 40*, 265–271.

Friebert, S.E., & Shurin, S.B. (1998). ALL: Diagnosis and outlook. *Contemporary Pediatrics, 15*(2), 118–136.

Furuta, T., Sugiu, K., Tamiya, T., Matsumoto, K., & Ohmoto, T. (1998). Malignant cerebellar astrocytoma developing 15 years after radiation therapy for a medulloblastoma [Review]. *Clinical Neurology and Neurosurgery, 100*, 56–59.

Gaddy-Cohen, D. (1993). Acute lymphocytic leukemia. In G.V. Foley, D. Fochtman, & K.H. Mooney (Eds.), *Nursing care of the child with cancer* (2nd ed.) (pp. 208–225). Philadelphia: W.B. Saunders.

Garaventa, A., DeBernardi, B., Pianca, C., Donfrancesco, A., diMontezemolo, L.C., DiTillio, M.T., Bagnulo, S., Mancini, A., Carli, M., Pession, A., Arrighini, A., DiCataldo, A., Tamaro, P., Iasonni, V., Taccone, A., Rogers, P., & Luca, B. (1993). Localized but unresectable neuroblastoma: Treatment and outcome of 145 cases. Italian Cooperative Group for Neuroblastoma. *Journal of Clinical Oncology, 11*, 1770–1779.

Giordana, M.T., Schiffer, P., & Schiffer, D. (1998). Prognostic factors in medulloblastoma. *Child's Nervous System, 14*, 256–262.

Golub, T.R., Weinstein, J.H., & Grier, H.E. (1997). Acute myelogenous leukemia. In P.A. Pizzo & D.G. Poplack (Eds.), *Principles and practice of pediatric oncology* (3rd ed.) (pp. 463–482). Philadelphia: Lippincott-Raven.

Graham, M.L., Herndon, J.E., III, Casey, J.R., Chaffee, S., Ciocci, G.H., Krischer, J.P., Kurtzberg, J., Laughlin, M.J., Longee, D.C., Olson, J.F., Paleologus, N., Pennington, C.M., & Friedman, H.S. (1997). High-dose chemotherapy with autologous stem cell rescue in patients with recurrent and high-risk pediatric brain tumors. *Journal of Clinical Oncology, 15*, 1814–1823.

Grimwade, D., Walker, H., Oliver, F., Wheatley, K., Harrison, C., Harrison, G., Rees, J., Hann, I., Stevens, R., Burnett, A., & Goldstone, A. (1998). The importance of diagnostic cytogenetics on outcome in AML: Analysis of 1,612 patients entered into the MRC AML 10 trial. *Blood, 92*, 2322–2333.

Guglielmi, M., DeBernardi, B., Rizzo, A., Siracusa, F., Leggio, A., Cozzi, F., Cecchetto, G., Musi, L., Bardini, T., Fagnani, A.M., Bartoli, G.C., Pampaloni, A., Rogers, D., Conte, M., Milanaccio, C., & Bruzzi, P. (1996). Resection of primary tumor at diagnosis in stage IV-S neuroblastoma: Does it affect the clinical course? *Journal of Clinical Oncology, 14*, 1537–1544.

Gurney, J.G., Severson, R.K., Davis, S., & Robison, L.L. (1995). Incidence of cancer in children in the United States. *Cancer, 75*, 2186.

Halligan, J.B., Stelzer, K.J., Rostomily, R.C., Spence, A.M., Griffin, T.W., & Berger, M.S. (1996). Operation and permanent low activity ^{125}I brachytherapy for recurrent high-grade astrocytomas. *International Journal of Radiation Oncology, Biology, Physics, 35*, 541–547.

Harris, M.B., Cantor, A.B., Goorin, A.M., Shochat, S.J., Ayala, A.G., Ferguson, W.S., Holbrook, T., & Link, M.P. (1995). Treatment of osteosarcoma with ifosfamide: Comparison of response in pediatric patients with recurrent disease versus patients previously untreated: A Pediatric Oncology Group study. *Medical and Pediatric Oncology, 24*, 87–92.

Harris, M.B., Shuster, J.J., Pullen, D.J., Borowitz, M.J., Carroll, A.J., Behm, F.G., & Land, V.J. (1998). Consolidation therapy with antimetabolite-based therapy in standard-risk acute lymphocytic leukemia of childhood: A Pediatric Oncology Group study. *Journal of Clinical Oncology, 16*, 2840–2847.

Heideman, R.L., Packer, R.J., Albright, L.A., Freeman, C.R., & Rorke, L.B. (1997). Tumors of the central nervous system. In P.A. Pizzo & D.G. Poplack (Eds.), *Principles and practice of pediatric oncology* (3rd ed.) (pp. 633–697). Philadelphia: Lippincott-Raven.

Hobbie, W., Ruccione, K., Moore, I., & Truesdell, S. (1993). Late effects in long-term survivors. In G.V. Foley, G. Fochtman, & K.H. Mooney (Eds.), *Nursing care of the child with cancer* (2nd ed.) (pp. 466–496). Philadelphia: W.B. Saunders.

Holcomb, G.W., Tomita, S.S., Haase, G.M., Dillon, P.W., Newman, K.D., Applebaum, H., & Wiener, E.S. (1995). Minimally invasive surgery in children with cancer. *Cancer, 76*, 121–128.

Horowitz, M.E., Malawer, M.M., Woo, S.Y., & Hicks, M. (1997). Ewing's sarcoma family of tumors: Ewing's sarcoma of bone and soft tissue and the peripheral primitive neuroectodermal tumors. In P.A. Pizzo & D.G. Poplack (Eds.), *Principles and practice of pediatric oncology* (3rd ed.) (pp. 831–863). Philadelphia: Lippincott-Raven.

Hudson, M.H., & Donaldson, S.S. (1997). Hodgkin's disease. In P.A. Pizzo & D.G. Poplack (Eds.), *Principles and practice of pediatric oncology* (3rd ed.) (pp. 523–543). Philadelphia: Lippincott-Raven.

Hurwitz, C.A., Mounce, K.G., & Grier, H.E. (1995). Treatment of patients with acute myelogenous leukemia: Review of clinical trials of the past decade. *Journal of Pediatric Hematology/Oncology, 17*, 185–197.

Hutchinson, R.J., Fryer, C.J., Davis, P.C., Nachman, J., Krailo, M.D., O'Brien, R.T., Collins, R.D., Whalen, T., Reardon, D., Trigg, M.E., & Gilchrist, G.S. (1998). MOPP or radiation in addition to ABVD in the treatment of pathologically staged advanced Hodgkin's disease in children. Results of the Children's Cancer Group phase III trial. *Journal of Clinical Oncology, 16*, 897–906.

Jarret, A.F., Armstrong, A.A., & Alexander, E. (1996). Epidemiology of EBV and Hodgkin's lymphoma. *Annals of Oncology, 7*(Suppl. 4), 5–10.

Jenkin, D. (1996). Long-term survival of children with brain tumors. *Oncology, 10*, 715–719.

Jennings, R.W., LaQuaglia, M.P., Leong, K., Hendren, W.H., & Adzick, N.S. (1993). Fetal neuroblastoma: Prenatal diagnosis and natural history. *Journal of Pediatric Surgery, 28*, 1168–1174.

Joshi, W., Cantor, A.B., Altshuler, G., Larkin, E.W., Neill, J.S., Shuster, J.J., Holbrook, C.T., Hayes, F.A., & Castleberry, R.P. (1992). Recommendations for modification of terminology of neuroblastic tumors and prognostic significance of Shimada classification. *Cancer, 69*, 2183–2196.

Kedar, A., Maria, B.L., Graham-Pole, J., Ringdahl, D.M., Quisling, R.G., Mickle, J.P., Mendenhall, N.P., Marcus, R.B., & Gross, S. (1994). High-dose chemotherapy with marrow reinfusion and hyperfractionated irradiation for children with high-risk brain tumors. *Medical and Pediatric Oncology, 23*, 428–436.

Khan, A.A., Villablanca, J.G., Reynolds, C.P., & Avramis, V.I. (1996). Pharmacokinetic studies of 13-cis-retinoic acid in pediatric patients with neuroblastoma following bone marrow transplantation. *Cancer Chemotherapy and Pharmacology, 39*, 1–2, 34–41.

Knudson, A.G., & Strong, L.C. (1972). Mutation and cancer: Neuroblastoma and pheochromocytoma. *American Journal of Human Genetics, 24*, 514–532.

Kuhl, J. (1998). Modern treatment strategies in medulloblastoma. *Child's Nervous System, 14*, 1–2, 25.

Kushner, B.H., Cheung, N.K., LaQuaglia, M.P., Ambros, P.F., Ambros, I.M., Bonilla, M.A., Ladanyi, M., & Gerald, W.L. (1996). International Neuroblastoma Staging System stage I neuroblastoma: A prospective study and literature review. *Journal of Clinical Oncology, 14*, 2174–2180.

Kushner, B.H., Gilbert, F., & Helson, L. (1986). Familial neuroblastoma. *Cancer, 57*, 1887–1893.

Kushner, B.H., LaQuaglia, M.P., Bonilla, M.A., Lindsley, K., Rosenfield, N., Yeh, S., Eddy, J., Gerald, W.L., Heller, G., & Cheung, N.K. (1994). Highly effective induction therapy for stage IV neuroblastoma in children over 1 year of age. *Journal of Clinical Oncology, 12*, 2607–2613.

Kushner, B.H., Meyers, P.A., Gerald, W.L., Healey, J.H., LaQuaglia, M.P., Boland, P., Wollner, N., Casper, E.S., Aledo, A., Heller, G., Schwartz, G.K., Bonilla, M.A., & Lindsley, K.L. (1995). Very-high-dose short-term chemotherapy for poor-risk peripheral primitive neuroectodermal tumors, including Ewing's sarcoma, in children and young adults. *Journal of Clinical Oncology, 13*, 2796–2804.

Landis, S.H., Murray, T., Bolden, S., & Wingo, P.A. (1999). Cancer statistics. *CA: A Cancer Journal for Clinicians, 49*, 8–31.

Link, M.P., & Eilber, F. (1997). Osteosarcoma. In P.A. Pizzo & D.G. Poplack (Eds.), *Principles and practice of pediatric oncology* (3rd ed.) (pp. 889–920). Philadelphia: Lippincott-Raven.

Link, M.P., Shuster, J.J., Donaldson, S.S., Berard, C.W., & Murphy, S.B. (1993). Treatment of children with localized non-Hodgkin's lymphoma (NHL) with nine weeks of chemotherapy with radiotherapy [Abstract]. *Medical and Pediatric Oncology, 21,* 532.

Lombardi, F., Navarria, P., & Gandola, L. (1998). The evolving role of radiation therapy in the optimal multimodality treatment of childhood cancer. *Tumori, 84,* 270–273.

Lukes, R.J., & Butler, J.J. (1966). The pathology and nomenclature of Hodgkin's disease. *Cancer Research, 26,* 1063.

Madero, L., Munoz, A., Sanches de Toledo, J., Diaz, M.W., Maldonado, M.S., Ortega, J.J., Ramirez, M., Otheo, E., Benito, A., & Salas, S. (1998). Megatherapy in children with high risk Ewing's sarcoma in first complete remission. *Bone Marrow Transplantation, 21,* 795–799.

Magrath, I., Adde, M., Shad, A., Venzon, D., Seibel, N., Gootenberg, J., Neely, J., Arndi, C., Nieder, M., Jaffe, E., Wittes, R.A., & Horak, I.D. (1996). Adults and children with small non-cleaved cell lymphoma have a similar excellent outcome when treated with the same chemotherapy regimen. *Journal of Clinical Oncology, 14,* 925–934.

Margolin, J.F., & Poplack, D.G. (1997). Acute lymphoblastic leukemia. In P.A. Pizzo & D.G. Poplack (Eds.), *Principles and practice of pediatric oncology* (3rd ed.) (pp. 409–462). Philadelphia: Lippincott-Raven.

Marina, N. (1997). Long-term survivors of childhood cancer—The medical consequences of cure. *Pediatric Clinics of North America, 44,* 1021–1042.

Mason, W.P., Grovas, A., Halpern, S., Dunkel, I., Garvin, J., Heller, G., Rosenblum, M., Gardner, S., Lyden, D., Sands, S., Puccetti, D., Lindsley, K., Merchant, T., O'Malley, B., Bayer, L., Petriccione, M., Allen, J., & Finlay, J. (1998). Intensive chemotherapy and bone marrow rescue for young children with newly diagnosed malignant brain tumors. *Journal of Clinical Oncology, 16,* 210–221.

Matthay, K.K., Perez, C., Seeger, R.C., Brodeur, G.M., Shimada, H., Atkinson, J.B., Black, C.T., Gerbing, R., Haase, G.M., Stram, D.O., Swift, P., & Lukens, J.N. (1998). Successful treatment of stage III neuroblastoma based on prospective biologic staging: A Children's Cancer Group study. *Journal of Clinical Oncology, 16,* 1256–1264.

McClain, K.L., Joshi, V.V., & Murphy, S.B. (1996). Cancers in children with HIV infection. *Hematology/Oncology Clinics of North America, 10,* 1189–1201.

McLaughlin, M.P., Marcus, R.B., Jr., Buatti, J.M., McCollough, W.M., Mickle, J.P., Kedar, A., Maria, B.L., & Million, R.R. (1998). Ependymoma: Results, prognostic factors and treatment recommendations. *International Journal of Radiation Oncology, Biology, Physics, 40,* 845–850.

Meyers, P.A., & Gorlick, R. (1997). Osteosarcoma. *Pediatric Clinics of North America, 44,* 973–989.

Meyers, P.A., Heller, G., Healey, J.H., Huvos, A., Applewhite, A., Sun, M., & LaQuaglia, M. (1993). Osteogenic sarcoma with clinically detectable metastasis at initial presentation. *Journal of Clinical Oncology, 11,* 449–453.

Moore, I.M. (1995). Central nervous system toxicity of cancer therapy in children. *Journal of Pediatric Oncology Nursing, 12,* 203–213.

Mueller, B.U., & Pizzo, P.A. (1997). Pediatric AIDS and childhood cancer. In P.A. Pizzo & D.G. Poplack (Eds.), *Principles and practice of pediatric oncology* (3rd ed.) (pp. 1005–1023). Philadelphia: Lippincott-Ravem.

Murphy, S.B., Fairclough, D.L., Hutchison, R.E., & Berard, C.W. (1989). Non-Hodgkin's lymphoma of childhood: An analysis of the histology, staging and response to treatment of 338 cases at a single institution. *Journal of Clinical Oncology, 7,* 186–193.

Mwanda, O.W., & Othierio-Abinya, H. (1998). Relapse of Hodgkin's disease after 10 years of complete remission: A case report. *East African Medical Journal, 75*(3), 192–194.

Nachman, J., Sather, H.N., Cherlow, J.M., Sensel, M.G., Gaynon, P.S., Lukens, J.N., Wolff, L., & Trigg, M.E. (1998). Response of children with high-risk acute lymphoblastic leukemia treated with and without cranial irradiation: A report from the Children's Cancer Group. *Journal of Clinical Oncology, 16,* 920–930.

Nachman, J., Sather, H.N., Gaynon, P.S., Lukens, J.N., Wolff, L., & Trigg, M.E. (1997). Augmented Berlin-Frankfurt-Munster therapy abrogates the adverse prognostic significance of slow early response to induction chemotherapy for children and adolescents with acute lymphoblastic leukemia and unfavorable presenting features: A report from the Children's Cancer Group. *Journal of Clinical Oncology, 15*, 2222–2230.

Needle, M.N., Molloy, P.T., Geyer, J.R., Herman-Liu, A., Belasco, J.B., Goldwein, J.W., Sutton, L., & Phillips, P.C. (1997). Phase II study of oral etoposide in children with recurrent brain tumors and other solid tumors. *Medical and Pediatric Oncology, 29*, 28–32.

Oberlin, O. (1996). Present and future strategies of treatment in childhood Hodgkin's lymphoma. *Annals of Oncology, 7*(Suppl. 4), 73–78.

Parker, B.R. (1997). Imaging studies in the diagnosis of pediatric malignancies. In P.A. Pizzo & D.G. Poplack (Eds.), *Principles and practice of pediatric oncology* (3rd ed.) (pp. 187–213). Philadelphia: Lippincott-Raven.

Petersen, F.B., Lynch, M.H., Clift, R.A., Applebaum, F.R., Sanders, J.E., Bensinger, W.I., Benyunes, M.C., Doney, K., Fefer, A., Martin, P., Stord, R., Rowley, S., Sullivan, K.M., Witherspoon, R., Weiden, P., Thomas, E.D., Fisher, L., Hansen, J.A., & Buckner, C.D. (1993). Autologous marrow transplantation for patients with acute myeloid leukemia in untreated first relapse or second complete remission. *Journal of Clinical Oncology, 11*, 1353–1360.

Petriccione, M.M. (1993). Central nervous system tumors. In G.V. Foley, G. Fochtman, & K.H. Mooney (Eds.), *Nursing care of the child with cancer* (2nd ed.) (pp. 239–253). Philadelphia: W.B. Saunders.

Pollack, I.F. (1994). Brain tumors in children. *New England Journal of Medicine, 331*, 1500–1507.

Prados, M.D., & Russo, C. (1998). Chemotherapy of brain tumors. *Seminars in Surgical Oncology, 14*(1), 88–98.

Prados, M.D., Berger, M.S., & Wilson, C.B. (1998). Primary central nervous system tumors: Advances in knowledge and treatment. *CA: A Cancer Journal for Clinicians, 48*, 331–360.

Provisor, A.J., Ettinger, L.J., Nachman, J.B., Krailo, M.D., Makley, J.T., Yunis, E.J., Huvos, A.G., Betcher, D.L., Baum, E.S., Kisker, C.T., & Miser, J.S. (1997). Treatment of nonmetastatic osteosarcoma of the extremity with pre-operative and post-operative chemotherapy: A report from the Children's Cancer Group. *Journal of Clinical Oncology, 15*, 76–84.

Pui, C-H., & Crist, W.M. (1994). Biology and treatment of acute lymphoblastic leukemia. *Journal of Pediatrics, 124*, 491–503.

Pui, C-H., & Evans, W.E. (1998). Acute leukemia. *New England Journal of Medicine, 339*, 605–615.

Pui, C-H., Evans, W.E., & Gilbert, J.R. (1998). Meeting report: International Childhood ALL Workshop. *Leukemia, 12*, 1313–1318.

Pui, C-H., Relling, M.V., Rivera, G.K., Hancock, M.L., Raimondi, S.C., Heslop, H.E., Santana, V.M., Ribeiro, R.C., Sandlund, J.T., Mahmoud, H.H., Evans, W.E., Crist, W.M., & Krance, R.A. (1995). Epipodophyllotoxin-related acute myeloid leukemia: A study of 35 cases. *Leukemia, 9*, 1990–1996.

Raimondi, S.C. (1993). Current status of cytogenetic research in childhood acute lymphoblastic leukemia. *Blood, 81*, 2237–2251.

Raney, R.B. (1997). Hodgkin's disease in childhood: A review. *Journal of Pediatric Hematology/Oncology, 19*, 502–509.

Raney, R.B., Asmar, L., Newton, W.A., Bagwell, C., Breneman, C., Crist, W., Gehan, E.A., Webber, B., Wharam, M., Wiener, E.S., Anderson, J.R., & Maurer, H.M. (1997). Ewing's sarcoma of soft tissues in childhood: A report from the Intergroup Rhabdomyosarcoma Study, 1972 to 1991. *Journal of Clinical Oncology, 15*, 574–582.

Ravindranath, Y., Abella, E., Krischer, J.P., Wiley, J., Inoue, S., Harris, M., Chauvenet, A., Alvarado, C.S., Dubowy, R., Ritchey, A.K., Land, V., Steuber, C.P., & Weinstein, H. (1992). Acute myeloid leukemia (AML) in Down's syndrome is highly responsive to chemotherapy: Experience on Pediatric Oncology Group AML study 8498. *Blood, 80*, 2210–2214.

Ravindranath, Y., Yeager, A.M., Change, M.N., Steuber, C.P., Krischer, J., Graham-Pole, J., Carrol, A., Inoue, S., Camitta, B., & Weinstein, H.J. (1996). Autologous bone marrow transplantation versus intensive consolidation chemotherapy for acute myeloid leukemia in childhood. Pediatric Oncology Group. *New England Journal of Medicine, 334*, 1428–1434.

Razzouk, B., Srinivas, S., Sample, C.E., Singh, V., & Sixbey, J.W. (1996). Epstein-Barr virus DNA recombination and loss in sporadic Burkitt's lymphoma. *Journal of Infectious Disease, 193*, 529–535.

Reiter, A., Schrappe, M., Panwaresch, R., Henze, G., Muller-Weihrich, S., Sauter, S., Sykora, K.W., Ludwig, W.D., Gadner, H., & Riehm, H. (1995). Non-Hodgkin's lymphomas of childhood and adolescence: Results of a treatment stratified for biologic subtypes and stage. A report of the Berlin-Frankfurt Munster Group. *Journal of Clinical Oncology, 13*, 359–372.

Ribeiro, R.C., Rivera, G.K., Hudson, M., Mulhern, R.K., Hancock, M.L., Kun, L., Mahmoud, H., Sandlund, J.T., & Crist, W.M. (1995). An intensive re-treatment protocol for children with an isolated CNS relapse of acute lymphoblastic leukemia. *Journal of Clinical Oncology, 13*, 333–338.

Robertson, P.L., Zeltzer, P.M., Boyett, J.M., Rorke, L.B., Allen, J.C., Geyer, J.R., Stanley, P., Li, H., Albright, A.L., McGuire-Cullen, P., Finlay, J.L., Stevens, K.R., Milstein, J.M., Packer, R.J., Wisoff, J., & the Children's Cancer Group. (1998). Survival and prognostic factors following radiation therapy and chemotherapy for ependymomas in children: A report of the Children's Cancer Group. *Journal of Neurosurgery, 88*, 695–670.

Robinson, L.L. (1997). General principles of the epidemiology of childhood cancer. In P.A. Pizzo & D.G. Poplack (Eds.), *Principles and practice of pediatric oncology* (3rd ed.) (pp. 1–10). Philadelphia: Lippincott-Raven.

Rubnitz, J.E., & Look, A.T. (1998). Molecular genetics of childhood leukemias. *Journal of Pediatric Hematology/Oncology, 20*, 1–11.

Russo, C., Cohn, S.L., Petruzzi, M.J., & deAlarcon, P.A. (1997). Long-term neurologic outcome in children with opsoclonus-myoclonus associated with neuroblastoma: A report from the Pediatric Oncology Group. *Medical and Pediatric Oncology, 28*, 284–288.

Saarinen, U., Wikstrom, S., Makipornaa, A., Lanning, M., Perkkio, M., Hovi, L., Rapola, J., & Sariola, H. (1996). In vivo purging of bone marrow in children with poor risk neuroblastoma for marrow collection and autologous bone marrow transplantation. *Journal of Clinical Oncology, 14*, 2791–2802.

Sanders, J., Glader, B., Cairo, M., Finkelstein, J.Z., Forman, E., Green, D., Luban, N., Bleyer, W.A., Lampkin, B.C., Murphy, S.B., & Woods, W.G. (1997). Guidelines for the pediatric cancer center and role of such centers in diagnosis and treatment: American Academy of Pediatrics Section Statement Section on Hematology/Oncology. *Pediatrics, 99*(1), 139–141.

Sandlund, J.T., Downing, J.R., & Crist, W.M. (1996). Non-Hodgkin's lymphoma in childhood. *New England Journal of Medicine, 334*, 1238–1248.

Sandlund, J.T., Pui, C-H., Santana, V.M., Mahmoud, H., Roberts, W.M., Morris, S., Raimondi, S., Ribeiro, R., Crist, W.M., Lin, J.S., Mao, L., Beraro, C.W., & Hutchison, R.E. (1994). Clinical features and treatment outcome for children with CD30+ large cell non-Hodgkin's lymphoma. *Journal of Clinical Oncology, 12*, 895–898.

Sawaya, R., Hammoud, M., Scmoppa, D., Hess, K.R., Wu, S.Z., Ski, W.M., & Wildrick, D.M. (1998). Neurosurgical outcomes in a modern series of 400 craniotomies for treatment of parenchymal tumors. *Neurosurgery, 42*, 1044–1055.

Schajowicz, F., Sissons, H.A., & Sobbin, L.H. (1995). The World Health Organization's histologic classification of bone tumors: A commentary on the second edition. *Cancer, 75*, 1208–1214.

Schellong, G. (1996). The balance between cure and late effects in childhood Hodgkin's lymphoma: The experience of the German–Austrian Pediatric Hodgkin's Disease Study Group since 1978. *Annals of Oncology, 7*(Suppl. 4), 67–72.

Scheurlen, W., & Kuhl, J. (1998). Current diagnostic and therapeutic management of CNS metastasis in childhood primitive neuroectodermal tumors and ependymomas. *Journal of Neuro-Oncology, 38,* 181–185.

Schmieglow, K., Glomstein, A., Kristinsson, J., Salmi, T., Schrode, R.H., & Bjork, O. (1997). Impact of morning versus evening schedule for oral methotrexate and 6-mercaptopurine on relapse risk for children with acute lymphoblastic leukemia. *Journal of Pediatric Hematology/Oncology, 19,* 102–109.

Scully, S.P., Temple, H.T., O'Keefe, R.J., Scarborough, M.T., Mankin, H.J., & Gebhardt, M.C. (1995). Role of surgical resection in pelvic Ewing's sarcoma. *Journal of Clinical Oncology, 13,* 2336–2341.

Shad, A., & Magrath, I.T. (1997). Malignant non-Hodgkin's lymphomas in children. In P.A. Pizzo & D.G. Poplack (Eds.), *Principles and practice of pediatric oncology* (3rd ed.) (pp. 545–587). Philadelphia: Lippincott-Raven.

Shankar, A.G., Ashley, S., Radford, M., Barrett, A., Wright, D., & Pinkerton, C.R. (1997). Does histology influence outcome in childhood Hodgkin's disease? Results from the United Kingdom Children's Cancer Study Group. *Journal of Clinical for Oncology, 15,* 2622–2630.

Shannon, K. (1998). Genetic predispositions and childhood cancer [Review]. *Environmental Health Perspectives, 1069*(Suppl. 3), 801–806.

Skarin, A.T., & Dorfman, D. (1997). Non-Hodgkin's lymphomas: Current classification and management. *CA: A Cancer Journal for Clinicians, 47,* 351–372.

Sklar, C.A. (1995). Growth following therapy for childhood cancer. *Cancer Investigations, 13,* 511–516.

Sklar, C.A. (1997). Growth and neuroendocrine dysfunction following therapy for childhood cancer. *Pediatric Clinics of North America, 44,* 489–503.

Steinherz, P.G., Gaynon, P.S., Breneman, J.E., Cherlow, J.M., Grossman, N.J., Kersey, J.H., Johnstone, H.S., Sather, H.N., Trigg, M.E., Chappell, R., Hammond, D., & Bieyer, W.A. (1996). Cytoreduction and prognosis in acute lymphoblastic leukemia. The importance of early marrow response: Report from the Children's Cancer Group. *Journal of Clinical Oncology, 14,* 389–398.

Sullivan, M.C. (1993). Neuroblastoma. In G.V. Foley, G. Fochtman, & K.H. Mooney (Eds.), *Nursing care of the child with cancer* (2nd ed.) (pp. 278–287) Philadelphia: W.B. Saunders.

Tabone, M.D., Kalifa, C., Rodary, C., Raquin, M., Valteau-Couanet, D., & Lemerle, J. (1994). Osteosarcoma recurrences in pediatric patients previously treated with intensive chemotherapy. *Journal of Clinical Oncology, 12,* 2614–2620.

Tallman, M.S., Anderson, J.W., Schiffer, C.A., Appelbaum, F.R., Frusner, J.H., Ogden, A., Shepherd, L., Willman, C., Bloomfield, C.D., Rowe, J.M., & Wiernik, P.M. (1997). All-trans-retinoic acid in acute promyelocytic leukemia. *New England Journal of Medicine, 337,* 1021–1028.

Taylor, A., Metcalfe, J.A., Thick, J., & Mak, Y.F. (1996). Leukemia and lymphoma in ataxia telangiectasia. *Blood, 87,* 423–438.

Tonini, G.P., Boni, L., Pession, A., Rogers, D., Iolascom, A., Basso, G., DiMontezemolo, L.C., Casale, F., Pession, A., Perri, P., Mazzocco, K., Scaruffi, P., LoCunsolo, C., Marchese, N., Milanaccio, C., Conte, M., Bruzzi, P., & DeBernardi, B. (1997). MYCN oncogene amplification in neuroblastoma is associated with worse prognosis, except in stage 4s: The Italian experience with 295 children. *Journal of Clinical Oncology, 15,* 85–93.

Tubergen, D.G., Krailo, M.D., Meadows, A.T., Rosenstock, J., Kadin, M., Morse, M., King, D., Steinherz, P.G., & Kersey, J.H. (1995). Comparison of treatment regimens for pediatric lymphoblastic non-Hodgkin's lymphoma: A Children's Cancer Group study. *Journal of Clinical Oncology, 13,* 1368–1376.

Uckun, F.M., Gaynon, P.S., Sather, H., Arthur, D., Trigg, M., Tubergen, D., Nachman, J., Steinherz, P., Sensel, M.G., & Reaman, G.R. (1997). Clinical features and treatment outcome of children with biphenotypic CD2$^+$, CD19$^+$ acute lymphoblastic leukemia: A Children's Cancer Group study. *Blood, 89,* 2488–2493.

Uckun, F.M., Gaynon, P.S., Sensel, M.G., Nachman, J., Trigg, M.E., Steinherz, P.G., Hutchinson, R., Bostrom, B.C., Sather, H.N., & Reaman, G.H. (1997). Clinical features and treatment outcome of childhood T-lineage acute lymphoblastic leukemia according to the apparent maturational stage of T-lineage leukemia blasts: A Children's Cancer Group study. *Journal of Clinical Oncology, 15*, 2214–2221.

Uckun, F.M., Steinherz, P.G., Sather, H., Trigg, M., Arthur, D., Tubergen, D., Gaynon, P., & Reamen, G. (1996). CD2 antigen expression on leukemic cells as a predictor of event free survival after chemotherapy for T cell lineage acute lymphoblastic leukemia: A Children's Cancer Group study. *Blood, 88*, 4288–4295.

Wartenburg, D. (1996). EMFs: Cutting through the controversy. *Public Health Reports, 111*(3), 204–217.

Weiner, L.A., Leventhal, B., Brecher, M.L., Marcus, R.B., Cantor, A., Gieser, P.W., Ternberg, J.L., Behm, F.G., Wharam, M.D., & Chauvenet, A.R. (1997). Randomized study of intensive MOPP-ABVD with or without low-dose total nodal radiation therapy in the treatment of stages IIB, IIIA2, IIIB, and IV Hodgkin's disease in pediatric patients: A Pediatric Oncology Group study. *Journal of Clinical Oncology, 15*, 2769–2779.

Wells, R.J., Woods, W.G., Buckley, J.D., Odom, L.F., Benjamin, D., Bernstein, J., Betcher, D., Feig, S., Kim, T., Ruymann, F., Smithson, W., Srivastava, A., Tannous, R., Buckley, C.M., Whitt, J.K., Wolff, L., & Lampkin, B.C. (1994). Treatment of newly diagnosed children and adolescents with acute myeloid leukemia: A Children's Cancer Group study. *Journal of Clinical Oncology, 12*, 2367–2377.

Wiley, F.M. (1993). Acute myelogenous leukemia. In G.V. Foley, G. Fochtman, & K.H. Mooney (Eds.), *Nursing care of the child with cancer* (2nd ed.) (pp. 226–234) Philadelphia: W.B. Saunders.

Woods, W.G., Tuchman, M., Robinson, L.L., Bernstein, M., Leclerc, J.M., Brisson, L.C., Brossard, J., Hill, G., Shurster, J., Luepker, R., Byrne, T., Weitzman, S., Bunin, G., & Lemieux, B. (1996). A population-based study of the usefulness of screening for neuroblastoma. *Lancet, 348*, 1682–1687.

Yaniv, I., Saab, A., Cohen, I.J., Goshen, Y., Lourn, D., Stark, B., Tamary, H., & Zaizov, R. (1996). Hodgkin's disease in children: Reduced tailored chemotherapy for stage I–II disease. *Journal of Pediatric Hematology/Oncology, 18*, 76–80.

Youmans, J.R. (Ed.). (1996). *Neurological surgery: A comprehensive reference guide to the diagnosis and management of neurosurgical problems* (4th ed.) (pp. 2493–3187). Philadelphia: W.B. Saunders.

CHAPTER 4.
The Survivorship Movement

Kathleen L. Neville, PhD, RN

Introduction

In recent years, the concept of survivorship has become a distinct reality for the increasing number of people who are living longer with cancer. More importantly, many now are cured of what were previously incurable and fatal diseases. Medical and technologic advances have dramatically improved survival rates of children and adolescents to greater than 60%. Meadows and Hobbie (1986) estimated that 1 of 1,000 young adults are survivors of pediatric cancer. More recent statistics cite a more favorable incidence. Bottomley (1998) stated that "by the year 2000, 1 of every 900 individuals ages 16–44 will be a survivor of childhood cancer" (p. 242).

Approximately 10 million people in the United States now include cancer as part of their medical history. Of these 10 million, 5,000 are estimated to have survived five years or more. Approximately 1,221,100 new cancer cases are estimated to be diagnosed in 2000 (American Cancer Society, 2000). The current five-year relative survival rate of all people with cancer is 59% (American Cancer Society). As medical science continues to progress, more and more people will become long-term survivors.

Scholarly journals, conference proceedings, and even media coverage have increasingly focused on the multitude of cancer survivorship issues across the life span. These issues have surfaced during the past decade as survivors began to voice their experiences of living with and beyond the cancer experience.

Defining Survivorship

Survivorship means different things to different people. Cure, recovery, and survivorship often are used synonymously when dealing with cancer, yet they are distinctly different. In the past, people with cancer were referred to as "victims of cancer." Today, they are referred to as "survivors of cancer." Before the curative capability of cancer treatment existed, "survivors of cancer" referred to surviving family members whose loved one died from cancer. When cancer treatment progressed to the point where the potential cure became a reality, physicians adopted the five-year parameter, which defined cancer survivors either from the time of diagnosis or the cessation of treatment (Leigh, 1992). In medicine, this usage of survivor still strongly applies, but other broad, all-encompassing definitions of survivorship exist.

Although survivorship is becoming a popular concept in oncology, further conceptual development is warranted (Leigh, 1992). Advances in the conceptual framework of survivorship can be achieved through a detailed concept analysis. A concept analysis is a highly useful approach to theory development and research in nursing and other related health disciplines that explores the attributes or characteristics of a concept. The process entails a careful examination of a word and the way it is used to impart meaning as well as how it is like or unlike similar terms (Walker & Avant, 1988). Through concept analysis, clarity can be achieved by removing the ambiguity in concepts of a theory or by providing a consistent definition of a term that is used frequently but, perhaps, not universally understood. Although a detailed concept analysis is not presented here, the term and its uses in the scientific literature are explored.

A conceptual definition is similar to a dictionary definition. Survive is defined as "to remain alive or in existence, after the death of another, or in spite of a mortally dangerous occurrence or situation" (Mish, 1996, p. 1186). Cancer survivorship refers to the unique state of living with the challenges of the cancer experience (Clark & Stovall, 1996). Rather than a stage in time, survivorship represents a process along a continuum and can be viewed as the experience of living with, through, and beyond cancer (Leigh, 1992). Survivorship does not represent a linear point in time; instead, it reflects a sense of movement through phases (Carter, 1989). Contrary to common understanding, survivorship is not synonymous with a benchmark time frame of cure. Instead, people with cancer are survivors beginning with the time of diagnosis and lasting for the remainder of their life (National Coalition for Cancer Survivorship [NCCS], 2000).

Survivorship Research

Survivorship is not a new research topic. Koocher and O'Malley's classic work (1981) describing the psychosocial consequences of surviving pediatric cancer and Mullan's (1985) classic work portraying the seasons of survival represent the foundational work of cancer survivorship. Healthcare professionals recognize the need to study the unique phenomenon of surviving cancer, which is now a research priority in cancer nursing (Fitch, 1996; Scott-Dorsett, 1991). But, what does the term survivorship imply? How is survivorship conceptualized? Clarity of these basic questions is necessary as scientists strive to improve the quality of life for increasing numbers of individuals who are diagnosed with cancer.

Fitzhugh Mullan, MD, cofounder of NCCS, wrote about his experience as a physician with cancer (1985). He described survival as an ill-defined but predictable condition through which all people with cancer pass as they struggle with their disease. All of the experiences of living with cancer characterize survival: the physical struggles of illness, surgery, and side effects of treatment; the mental struggles of fear, anxiety, and uncertainty; the overall disruption of life; and all of the normal life experiences that occur regardless of illness. He described the three seasons of survival as acute, extended, and permanent. The acute season of survival represents the medical phase that begins at diagnosis and centers on treatment modalities. The extended season of survival represents the time of remission or completion of the basic treatment regimen that is marked by less frequent periodic health examinations or contact with the oncology healthcare team. The last season, permanent survival, is comprised of several dimensions, including what commonly is referred to as cure. Mullan stated that "there is no moment of cure but, rather, an evolution from the phase of extended survival into a period when the activity of the disease or the likelihood of its return is sufficiently small that the cancer can now be considered permanently arrested" (p. 272). A range of individuals can experience long-term survivorship, from those living with persistent but medically controlled disease to those who are free of disease (Welch-McCaffrey, Hoffman, Leigh, Loescher, & Meyskens, 1989).

The Experience of Anomia

In an exploratory study of people recovering from cancer, Maher (1982) described the negative aspects of recovery and applied the concept of anomia to the recovery experience. Anomia is defined as "a temporary state of mind, occasioned by a sudden alteration in one's life situation and characterized by confusion, anxiety, uncertainty, loss of purpose, and sense of separation from one's usual social support system" (p. 911).

Completion of treatment and fear of possible recurrence create anxiety and uncertainty in people. Although healthcare professionals generally view long periods of time without recurrence as favorable, Maher asserted that people with cancer may hold a different view. By avoiding use of the word "cured," people are aware of the potential for recurrence. As time passes, the possibility that the disease is not cured becomes more threatening, and people may feel that time is running out.

Indeterminacy is another element of anomia regarding cancer survival. When faced with cancer, healthcare professionals use a "one day at a time" approach to counsel patients and their family members on matters of dealing with cancer and its treatment. Beginning at diagnosis, patients and their families are encouraged to shift from future-oriented behavior to a present-day orientation of life. In modern-day living, however, identity and self-concept are entwined with future goals and expectations. Until the time when future orientation is reestablished, people's self-concept and identity are of an indeterminate nature. Burdened with the realities of potential job discrimination, prolonged absence from work, alteration in energy level, and role changes in the family and work environment, people may be unable to fully appreciate the good fortune of surviving cancer. Additionally, one of the critical aspects of anomia regarding recovery from cancer is the loss or reduction of social support after treatment ends. When people are no longer acutely ill, family members and other supportive people often feel depleted of energy and anxious to regain a semblance of normalcy in their lives (Neville, 1996). Unfortunately, people still may be feeling very traumatized by the cancer experience and are left to sort out the whole ordeal alone. Complete rehabilitation of patients with cancer is not achieved until they are provided with the opportunity to "talk through" the experience with people who can appreciate the new meaning it has imparted on life (Maher, 1982).

A phenomenological study exploring the lived experience of having cancer described similar findings (Hallsdorsdottir & Hamrin, 1996). In-depth interviews with people in the remission or recovery phase identified existential changes as the major theme of analysis. The five subthemes of existential changes were uncertainty, vulnerability, discomfort, isolation, and redefinition of self.

The Growing Voice of Survivors

Survivors' voices now are being heard loud and clear, largely because of NCCS. This grass roots network developed from the vision of 25 leaders and experts in cancer research, community-based support services, information services, and advocacy. This group met in Albuquerque, NM, in 1986 and founded an organization of, by, and for cancer survivors. "Through thoughtful and responsible advocacy, NCCS has assumed a leadership role in the survivorship movement and the cancer community" (NCCS, 1998, p. 3). The organization's vision is that all people with cancer will receive as much information as possible about their treatment options to ensure the best quality of life. More importantly, NCCS proposes that all people will have equal opportunity to access treatment and support services. Its mission is "to ensure quality cancer care for all Americans," and its goals are "to lead and strengthen the survivorship movement, to empower cancer survivors, and to advocate for policy issues that affect cancer survivors' quality of life" (NCCS, 2000).

NCCS publications address the vitally important issue of the need for increased funding for cancer research, which is reflected in sobering statistics. Approximately 1,500 people die of cancer each day in the United States, whereas approximately 496,000 Americans have died in the five wars fought in this century. A startling 550,000 Americans die of cancer every year, but only one penny from every $10 paid in taxes goes toward fighting cancer (NCCS, 1998). NCCS's strong efforts are directed toward making changes in the healthcare system that will lead to a higher number of cancer survivors.

The March

On September 26, 1998, in Washington, DC, NCCS held "The March: Coming Together to Conquer Cancer," the culmination of an 18-month national public awareness and grass roots organizing campaign. Numerous cancer-related organizations endorsed the gathering in an effort to present a united front against cancer. Politicians, sports figures, entertainers, celebrities, and family members spoke about the impact of cancer on their lives. During the weekend of "The March," NCCS held a vigil and interfaith service to honor survivors and remember people who died of cancer. Two large screens displayed an honor roll of names and pictures of people who died of cancer. A sea of lighted candles represented the incredible number of people whose lives have been affected by cancer. Numerous educational displays, children's activities, health fairs, rallies, and benefits were held in conjunction with the event. The mission of "The March" was to make cancer America's top research priority, to demand more attention to all cancer research, to ensure equal access to quality care for all Americans, and to put "public" back into public policy decisions (NCCS, 1998).

Self-Advocacy

NCCS strongly endorses the value of peer support, advocacy, and empowerment in dealing with the numerous issues involved with surviving cancer. Kohnke (1980) first described advocacy in nursing in terms of providing information to educate and support individuals to enable them to make the best decisions possible for themselves. One of the most important messages that NCCS communicates to people who are diagnosed with cancer is that they are not alone. A tremendous network of support is available to them. Support groups are also valuable to survivors because they need to learn to advocate for themselves. The caring and concern of others facilitate this process. Although each individual has a unique experience with cancer, threads of universality exist. People who share their stories help themselves and others to survive cancer. Self-advocacy leads to the autonomy of making informed choices. Advocacy emphasizes a competency model of survivorship that focuses on building skills and developing effective coping strategies (Clark & Stovall, 1996).

Many benefits of self-advocacy in cancer survivorship have been cited. According to Stovall and Clark (1996), advocacy provides people with a sense of stability and control in life, confidence to face challenges, improved quality of life, feelings of hopefulness rather than hopelessness, and a way of reaching out to others.

Self-advocacy provides people with the necessary resources to make the best decisions for themselves. Peer support and self-help groups can be invaluable resources to learn self-advocacy. Support groups became incredibly popular in the 1980s. Today, support groups exist for people with all types of health conditions. These groups provide education and links to other resources for information and treatment. More importantly, the group experience allows people to communicate, share, and normalize their experiences with illness. Clark and Stovall (1996) identified the need for cancer survivorship skills training to help people to deal with the multiple issues of cancer. Problem-solving skills are essential to successfully manage the complex cancer experience. Accurate information is the foundation of problem solving, and information needs will change throughout the course of an illness. For instance, during the diagnostic period, patients need information about their cancer, the treatment, anticipated limitations in their previous activities, and side effects.

After treatment, patients need information about the physical and psychosocial sequelae. Reintegration issues (i.e., moving from "patient" back to "person") also need to be addressed. Survivors of cancer need to be able to seek information from healthcare providers, and, in many cases, this is a learned skill.

Throughout the past three decades, healthcare delivery has undergone an incredible shift toward a patient-centered approach and open communication in cancer care. In the 1960s, doctors and families normally withheld information from patients regarding a cancer diagnosis. Based on the assumption that patients were better off not knowing about a grave prognosis, this lack of disclosure was believed to benefit patients. This "conspiracy of silence" lost favor in the United States in the 1970s as physicians who were working with patients with cancer found that the use of open communication enhanced their patients' sense of trust and created a stronger rapport (Holland, 1990). Unfortunately, in other cultures, patients still are denied information regarding their health status and full disclosure is not afforded to patients faced with cancer. A tremendous movement in healthcare-related consumerism that began in the 1970s has resulted in the availability of numerous publications that help people to communicate with healthcare professionals when seeking health care.

A cancer diagnosis is a crisis situation. Good problem-solving skills are crucial when making potentially life-altering decisions, often at a time when cognitive processes may be impaired as a result of stress or physiologic injury. Problem-solving skills that focus on choices, alternatives, decision-making processes, and ways to initiate action are absolutely vital to making responsible decisions in a crisis. Stovall and Clark (1996) reported that negotiation skills are often necessary in dealing with cancer survivorship. Not only is advocacy necessary for receiving appropriate health care, but survivors also must advocate for medical benefits and legal rights. Although state and federal laws exist to protect survivors from job discrimination, many survivors still report difficulties in finding and maintaining employment. Negotiating skills are a valuable asset to survivors who may have to change their employment or vocation or self-advocate for new training. Assertiveness is now a necessary skill for survivors of cancer and marks a dramatic change in patient-physician relationships from the past. Unlike years ago, patients facing cancer today are no longer passive recipients of care but are active participants who interact, offer input, and mutually participate with healthcare professionals. The concept of empowerment is important to this view of self-advocacy. Empowerment refers to the process of influencing others that affect one's life. People who describe themselves as empowered believe that they are capable of understanding their own needs better than others can (Stovall & Clark). As part of the growing survivorship movement, the American Cancer Society published the Cancer Survivor's Bill of Rights in 1998 (see Figure 4-1). In addition, NCCS formulated the Quality Cancer Care Declaration of Principles, which was adopted at the First National Congress on Cancer Survivorship in 1995.

Common Issues of Survivorship

Given the relatively recent advances in science that have altered or lengthened the life span of many patients with cancer, many of the issues that cancer survivors face are relatively new. Common

---

Figure 4-1. The Cancer Survivor's Bill of Rights

1. Survivors have the right to assurance of lifelong medical care, as needed. The physicians and other professionals involved in their care should continue their constant efforts to be:
   - Sensitive to the cancer survivors' lifestyle choices and their need for self-esteem and dignity;
   - Careful, no matter how long they have survived, to take symptoms seriously, and not have aches and pains dismissed, for fear of recurrence is a normal part of survivorship;
   - Informative and open, providing survivors with as much or as little candid medical information as they wish, and encouraging their informed participation in their own care;
   - Knowledgeable about counseling resources, and willing to refer survivors and their families as appropriate for emotional support and therapy which will improve the quality of individual lives.
2. In their personal lives, survivors, like other Americans, have the right to the pursuit of happiness. This means they have the right:
   - To talk with their families and friends about their cancer experiences if they wish, but to refuse to discuss it if that is their choice and not to be expected to be more upbeat or less blue than anyone else;
   - To be free of the stigma of cancer as a "dread disease" in all social relations;
   - To be free of blame for having gotten the disease and guilt of having survived it.
3. In the work place, survivors have the right to equal job opportunities. This means they have the right:
   - To aspire to jobs worthy of their skills, and for which they are trained and experienced, and thus not have to accept jobs they would not have considered before the cancer experience;
   - To be hired, promoted, and accepted on return to work, according to their individual abilities and qualifications, and not according to "cancer" or "disability" stereotypes.
   - To privacy about their medical histories.
4. Since health insurance coverage is an overriding survivorship concern, every effort should be made to assure all survivors adequate health insurance, whether public or private. This means:
   - For employers, that survivors have the right to be included in group health coverage, which is usually less expensive, provides better benefits, and covers the employee regardless of health history;
   - For physicians, counselors, and other professionals concerned, that they keep themselves and their survivor-clients informed and up-to-date on available group or individual health policy options, noting, for example, what major expenses like hospital costs and medical tests outside the hospital are covered and what amount must be paid before coverage (deductible).
   - For social policy makers, both in government and in the private sector, that they seek to broaden insurance programs like Medicare to include diagnostic procedures and treatment which help prevent recurrence and ease survivor anxiety and pain.

Note. Written by Natalie Davis Springarn and published in *A Cancer Survivor's Almanac: Charting Your Journey*, copyright © 1996 National Coalition for Cancer Survivorship. Used by permission.

issues related to survivorship entail long-term or late physiologic effects, job discrimination and stigma, fatigue, anxiety, and depression.

Long-Term Physiologic Effects

Advanced modern multimodality treatment plans have dramatically improved survival rates. These combined treatment modalities that destroy cancer cells also can destroy or damage healthy cells and organs. Unfortunately, people who are treated successfully also are at risk for the medical complications of their treatment modalities. Long-term effects are known or expected medical problems that can occur months to many years after completion of treatment and occur with some frequency in people who have undergone certain treatments (Ganz, 1998). Long-term effects are secondary conditions that occur as a direct result of treatment.

Data on the long-term and late effects of cancer treatment now are being gathered. Since the beginning cures of cancer, which were seen in children diagnosed with acute lymphocytic leukemia, testicular cancer, and Hodgkin's disease, long-term effects have been identified and recognized for a greater length of time in the pediatric population. Findings from earlier survivors changed pediatric protocols. The goal of eradicating disease with the least amount of treatment minimizes the long-term and late effects of treatment that children and adolescents experience.

These late effects may be very varied, very obvious, or very subtle. They can range from overt impairment of activities of daily living, cognitive dysfunction, and memory impairment to subclinical findings that only screening and testing reveal.

Organ toxicity is a real possibility, particularly when certain chemotherapeutic agents and radiation are used (see Figure 4-2). Cardiotoxicity is associated most frequently with mediastinal radiation and high-dose daunorubicin, doxorubicin, and cyclophosphamide (Ganz, 1998). However, Hobbie, Ruccione, Moore, and Truesdell (1993) reported isolated cases of cardiovascular complications in patients who received low doses of these chemotherapeutic agents. Anthracycline-induced cardiovascular abnormalities are observed in approximately 25% of patients (Hobbie et al.). When mediastinal radiation is combined with these agents, cardiac abnormalities may occur with even lower doses (Ganz). The long-term effects of childhood and adolescent cancer treatment can occur during periods of cardiovascular stress (e.g., vigorous exercise, pregnancy, weight lifting, illness, substance abuse) (Ganz; Hobbie et al.). Long-term survivors who received mantle radiation (e.g., children and adolescents with Hodgkin's disease) can experience premature coronary artery disease.

Acute and chronic pulmonary toxicities also are associated with cancer treatment. Acute pneu-

Figure 4-2. Organ Systems and Tissues at Risk for Late Toxicity From Cancer Treatment

- Bone and soft tissues
- Cardiovascular
- Dental
- Endocrine
- Gastrointestinal
- Hepatic
- Hematologic
- Immunologic
- Nervous system
- Neuropsychological
- Ophthalmologic
- Pulmonary
- Renal
- Reproductive

Note. From "Cancer Survivors: Physiologic and Psychosocial Outcomes" (p. 119) by P.A. Ganz in M.C. Perry (Ed.), *American Society of Clinical Oncology Spring Educational Book*, 1998, Chestnut Hill, MA: Author. Copyright 1998 by the American Society of Clinical Oncology. Reprinted with permission.

monitis usually occurs three to six months after radiation treatment. Chronic pulmonary fibrosis occurs later, clinically presenting as dyspnea, dry cough, and exercise intolerance that frequently progress with aging. The chemotherapeutic agents bleomycin, nitrosoureas, and busulfan can cause chronic pulmonary fibrosis. Renal damage can occur after treatment with several different chemotherapeutic agents or radiation therapy. Acute and chronic nephrotoxicity is associated with cisplatin, methotrexate, and nitrosoureas (Ganz, 1998). Other effects on the urinary tract include cystitis, urethral strictures, and enuresis. Cancer treatment may markedly affect the growth and development of children and adolescents. Aside from the endocrine effects of treatment, radiation therapy affects growing bones, soft tissues, and epiphyses and dramatically affects growth (Hobbie et al., 1993).

Scoliosis, kyphosis, and shortened sitting height are sequelae of irradiation to the vertebral bodies. Because of the combination of steroids and radiation used to treat Hodgkin's and non-Hodgkin's lymphoma, avascular necrosis of the femoral head may occur. Radiation can damage the growth plates of long bones and cause muscle atrophy, osteonecrosis, and fractures (Ganz, 1998). Chronic pain may occur as a result of scarring and fibrosis of soft tissues surrounding nerves and joints that have received radiation (Ganz).

If children or adolescents receive radiation to the head and neck region, maxillofacial abnormalities frequently occur. Malocclusion, poor root and enamel formation, and decreased salivary function, which may predispose patients to the development of dental caries, may occur (Ganz, 1998; Hobbie et al., 1993).

Substantial neurologic complications can occur in children and adolescents who have been treated for cancer. Cranial irradiation and intrathecal chemotherapy can result in cognitive impairment. Manifestations of cognitive impairment include a decline in academic achievement tests and varying degrees of memory loss. Deficits in abstract reasoning, motor skills, visual-spatial abilities, and concentration skills also can be evident. Peripheral neuropathies are not uncommon and can be particularly disabling. Children treated for leukemia with central nervous system prophylaxis are most vulnerable to cognitive impairment.

Hematologic and immunologic dysfunction are common during and shortly after treatment, but, in some cancers, permanent changes in function may occur. With Hodgkin's lymphoma, immunologic impairment may be both a result of treatment and part of the disease itself. Patients who have undergone a splenectomy are at increased risk for serious bacterial infections. Radiation to the bone marrow or chemotherapy can result in myelosuppression.

Numerous endocrine system problems can occur from cancer treatment. These problems are either the result of damage to the hypothalamus and pituitary region or to the end organ (e.g., ovaries, testes, thyroid) (Hobbie et al., 1993). Treating children with radiation to the head can cause growth hormone deficiencies and even retardation. Precocious puberty has been identified in children who have received radiation to the hypothalamus (Hobbie et al.).

Children and adolescents who have received radiation treatment to the head and neck are at risk for hypothyroidism following direct radiation to the thyroid gland. A secondary hypothyroidism may occur in patients who receive radiation to the hypothalamic-pituitary axis (Hobbie et al., 1993).

Gonadal dysfunction or failure is of particular concern for children and adolescents with cancer. Cancer-related treatment can cause male and female infertility, impaired libido, halted pubertal development, and impaired secondary sex characteristics that can dramatically affect body image and psychological adjustment. Young girls who receive radiation to the abdominal cavity may later experience miscarriage secondary to a decrease in uterine capacity (Ganz, 1998). Visual and hearing impairment also can occur after cancer treatment. Cisplatin administration can cause hearing deficit, particularly inability to hear high-pitched sounds. Radiation directed to the auditory system also can result in hearing impairment. Radiation to the eye can be very damaging and may cause cataract formation. Table 4-1 lists possible late effects of radiotherapy, Table 4-2 lists the late effects of chemotherapy, and Table 4-3 lists the late effects of surgery.

Secondary malignancies are perhaps the most feared potential complications. People who have survived a malignancy and been treated with chemotherapy and radiation are at an increased risk for developing secondary tumors. Specific cancers and their concomitant treatment pose specific risks. For instance, adolescents who are diagnosed with Hodgkin's disease are at an increased risk for developing breast and thyroid cancer as a result of radiation treatment. Patients being treated with cytoxan are at an increased risk for developing bladder cancer. Knowledge gained throughout the past two decades from studying survivors of cancer has led to methods for early detection of secondary malignancies. Data obtained from present-day and future survivors undoubtedly will create changes in treatment modalities and hopefully reduce the morbidity and mortality of cancer treatment sequelae.

Job Discrimination

Despite laws that protect against discrimination, many survivors report job discrimination as a result of their cancer experience. Survivors most often report dismissal, failure to hire, demotion, denial of promotion, unfair transfer, hostility, and denial of benefits (Hoffman, 1996). Although anyone can experience discrimination, Hoffman identified that certain groups are particularly at

Table 4-1. Possible Late Effects of Radiotherapy

Organ System	Late Effects/Sequelae
All tissues	Secondary malignancies
Bone and soft tissues	Abnormal growth and short stature, atrophy, fibrosis, cosmetic deformities
Dental/oral health	Poor enamel formation, poor root formation, dry mouth
Ophthalmologic	Cataracts, keratoconjunctivitis, retinopathy
Cardiovascular	Pericardial effusion, constrictive pericarditis, premature coronary artery disease
Pulmonary	Pulmonary fibrosis, decreased lung volume
Central nervous system	Neuropsychological deficits, structural changes, hemorrhage
Hematologic	Cytopenia, myelodysplasia
Renal	Hypertension, decreased creatinine clearance
Genitourinary	Bladder fibrosis, contractures
Gastrointestinal	Malabsorption, intestinal stricture, abnormal liver function
Endocrine	Growth hormone deficiency, other signs of pituitary deficiency
Thyroid	Hypothyroidism (overt or compensated), thyroid nodules
Gonadal	Men: risk of sterility, Leydid cell dysfunction; Women: ovarian failure, possible early menopause

Note. From "Cancer Survivors: Physiologic and Psychosocial Outcomes" (p. 120) by P.A. Ganz in M.C. Perry (Ed.), *American Society of Clinical Oncology Spring Educational Book*, 1998, Chestnut Hill, MA: Author. Copyright 1998 by the American Society of Clinical Oncology. Reprinted with permission.

Table 4-2. Possible Late Effects of Chemotherapy

Organ System	Drug	Late Effects/Sequelae
Bone	Corticosteroids	Avascular necrosis
Cardiopulmonary	Anthracycline High-dose cyclophosphamide Bleomycin Methotrexate Carmustine Actinomycin D/doxorubicin	Cardiomyopathy, congestive heart failure Congestive heart failure Pulmonary fibrosis Interstitial pneumonitis Pulmonary fibrosis Potentiate radiation effects
Ophthalmologic	Corticosteroids	Cataracts
Central nervous system and peripheral nervous system	Methotrexate Cisplatin Vinca alkaloids, paclitaxel	Possible structural changes, neuropsychiatric changes, hemiplegia, seizures Peripheral neuropathy, hearing loss Peripheral neuropathy
Renal	Cisplatin Methotrexate Nitrosoureas	Decreased creatinine clearance, magnesium wasting Increased creatinine, renal failure Delayed onset renal failure
Genitourinary	Cyclophosphamide	Hemorrhagic cystitis, bladder fibrosis
Hematologic	Alkylating agents	Myelodyplastic syndromes
Gastrointestinal	Methotrexate Carmustine	Abnormal liver function tests, hepatic fibrosis, cirrhosis Abnormal liver function tests, hepatic failure
Gonadal	Alkylating agents Procarbazine	Men: sterility; Women: sterility, premature menopause

Note. From "Cancer Survivors: Physiologic and Psychosocial Outcomes" (p. 120) by P.A. Ganz in M.C. Perry (Ed.), *American Society of Clinical Oncology Spring Educational Book,* 1998, Chestnut Hill, MA: Author. Copyright 1998 by the American Society of Clinical Oncology. Reprinted with permission.

Table 4-3. Late Effects of Surgery

Procedure	Late Effect
Amputation	Functional changes, cosmetic deformity, psychosocial impact
Abdominal surgery	Risk of intestinal obstruction
Lymphadenectomy	Lymphedema
Splenenctomy	Impaired immune function, risk of sepsis from encapsulated organisms
Pelvic surgery	Impotence, incontinence

Note. From "Cancer Survivors: Physiologic and Psychosocial Outcomes" (p. 120) by P.A. Ganz in M.C. Perry (Ed.), *American Society of Clinical Oncology Spring Educational Book,* 1998, Chestnut Hill, MA: Author. Copyright 1998 by the American Society of Clinical Oncology. Reprinted with permission.

risk. Nonprofessional or blue-collar employees have more problems with job discrimination than professional or white-collar. Survivors of childhood cancer have greater difficulty obtaining insurance policies for health, life, and disability through the workplace, have slightly lower incomes, and have fewer opportunities in military service than other young adults (Hoffman).

The Americans With Disabilities Act (ADA), passed in 1990, prohibits some types of job discrimination by employers, labor unions, and employment agencies against people who have had or have cancer. ADA defines cancer as a disability, regardless of status (i.e., cured, in remission, or not responsive to treatment) (Hoffman, 1996), and prohibits discrimination against people with any disability. This federal act requires employers to treat all employees similarly and to make reasonable accommodations for people during or after cancer treatment. Prior to this law, the Federal Rehabilitation Act was the only federal law that prohibited discrimination against cancer survivors. This act prohibits public and private employers who receive public funds from discriminating on the basis of a disability (Hoffman).

In 1993, President Clinton signed the Family and Medical Leave Act, which provides job security to people who must tend to the illness-related needs of themselves or a family member. In organizations of 50 or more employees, the Family and Medical Leave Act provides job protection by allowing a maximum of 12 weeks of unpaid leave during the treatment and recovery period. This act is very important to cancer survivors because employers must continue to provide health benefits during this leave period.

Despite massive public education efforts, the myths of cancer as a contagion still pervade and stigmatize some people. Recently, however, survivors have won cancer discrimination cases. Cancer survivors' knowledge of their legal rights is increasingly becoming a major component of self-advocacy.

Education Issues for Children and Adolescents With Cancer

Because long-term survival is now a realistic outcome for many children and adolescents with cancer, the importance of their education process is increasingly being recognized. Because of scientific advances, the focus of comprehensive care of children and adolescents with cancer has expanded from mere survival of a potentially life-threatening illness to survival as a fully functioning, productive member of society (Deasy-Spinetta, 1997). Children and adolescents with cancer not only need physiologic and psychological care, but social and academic development also must be considered.

Children or adolescents with cancer should return to school as soon as medically possible after the initial diagnosis (Deasy-Spinetta, 1997). The benefits of early return are significant: children are allowed to experience normalization, and, after the crisis of diagnosis, their equilibrium is restored and a sense of self returns (Deasy-Spinetta). In addition, children and adolescents are spared the ambiguity regarding whether they will return to school.

Role clarification is necessary for all of the people who are facilitating and supporting the education opportunities of children or adolescents with cancer. The parents' primary role is advocate. Their role involves communicating effectively with the various members of the education and medical team (e.g., school nurses, principals, teachers, physicians, social workers, guidance counselors). Effective communication is necessary to eliminate unnecessary fears and myths that may exist because of inadequate knowledge and education and to dispel any rumors regarding a child or adolescent's condition. The school liaison is in a prime position to support the parents by informing them of what to tell the school, how to speak with teachers, how to screen for communicable diseases, and how to manage the negative reactions of other children (e.g., teasing, harassing).

The school is primarily responsible for educating children and adolescents. Rather than focusing on the illness, attention should focus on academic background. Although school personnel need medical information regarding health status to plan for education needs, the primary emphasis should be on education. Previous academic and social achievement level prior to illness should be assessed. A treatment plan, modified from that baseline level, then needs to be devised. Children and adolescents in school must remain students and not be labeled patients. The school also is responsible for facilitating peer, faculty, and staff education regarding a child's or adolescent's disease and, specifically, factors affecting attendance, peer and social interaction, education, and medical compliance.

Unique education needs must be met for adolescents with cancer to obtain the common goals of securing employment or attending college after high school. To meet either goal, planned education intervention is necessary to ensure that adolescents meet their education requirements. In addition, assessment and evaluation of disease and treatment sequelae and its impact on learning and career choice alternatives are necessary. Job placement, counseling, and rehabilitation may be needed. The ultimate task of the multidisciplinary education and healthcare team is to promote maximum independence, autonomy, self-worth, and accomplishment in survivors of childhood or adolescent cancer. However, not all children and adolescents with cancer need special education or other services. These children and adolescents should be allowed to continue school without any modifications and, if necessary, should receive short-term home instruction. Advances in education technology (e.g., Internet, teledistance learning) offer invaluable options for students to continue their academic studies outside of the classroom.

Many disease- and treatment-related effects negatively affect the academic potential of some children and adolescents. Numerous special services are available to assess and evaluate cognitive, language, physical, speech, psychosocial, and developmental disabilities as well as to provide intervention. Just as laws exist to protect adults from discrimination, laws exist to protect children and adolescents. Acts also exist that provide for education and vocation training and career development.

Three federal legislative acts protect the rights of children and adolescents with cancer. The Individuals with Disabilities Education Act enables students with disabilities to receive special education and related services. The Federal Rehabilitation Act, which prohibits federal agencies, contractors, and those who are recipients of federal aid from discriminating against disabled individuals, also prohibits discrimination in employment, preschool through postsecondary education, and nonacademic and extracurricular activities (e.g., health and counseling services, clubs, transportation) (Deasy-Spinetta, 1997). The ADA prohibits discrimination against people with disabilities. Unlike the Federal Rehabilitation Act, the ADA applies to private and state organizations, not just federal agencies.

Future Research

Since its inception, NCCS has advocated for more cancer survivorship research. The National Cancer Institute established the Office of Cancer Survivorship (OCS), whose mission is to identify and prioritize the future cancer survivorship research agenda (Meadows, 1998). OCS identified many of the problems that cancer survivors face and named the following as priority areas needing more research: quality of life; physiologic outcomes; reproductive and sexuality issues; secondary malignancies; patient education, communication, and intervention; economic outcomes; and new data resources to comprehensively address survivorship issues (Meadows).

Quality of life is an important factor of long-term survivorship, yet much of the research has focused on quality of life only during the treatment phase. Longitudinal studies are needed, with measurements that tap issues of employment, insurance, and sexuality (Meadows, 1998). Investigations regarding the frequency and types of adverse physiologic outcomes are necessary. Treatment can profoundly affect sexuality, reproduction, and quality of life. Sexuality and reproductive outcomes are especially important for children or adolescents with cancer, particularly regarding reproductive capability and the effect of treatment on offspring. Data on the high incidence of secondary malignancies already exist, but the factors that increase risk need to be determined and quantified (Meadows). The specific information needs of cancer survivors must be identified through research. Research needs to be conducted on primary care physicians' and specialists' knowledge of cancer survivorship, how they conduct follow-up practices, and how they convey information to survivors. Research needs to focus on understanding how the underserved and at-risk populations perceive care and to determine the overall differences in their treatment experience compared to mainstream society or those with financial and/or insurance coverage. Lastly, the economic issues of cancer need to be investigated because cost-containment is and will remain a large determinant in the provision of cancer care. Indirect costs of cancer survivorship (e.g., lost wages and work, disability, the cost of long-term complications) also need to be studied (Meadows).

References

American Cancer Society. (2000). *Cancer facts & figures, 2000*. Atlanta: Author.

Bottomley, S. (1998). Late effects of childhood cancer. In M.J. Hockenberry-Eaton (Ed.), *Essentials of pediatric oncology nursing: A core curriculum* (pp. 241–274). Glenview, IL: Association of Pediatric Oncology Nurses.

Carter, B. (1989). Going through: A critical theme in surviving breast cancer. *Innovations in Oncology Nursing, 5*, 2–4.

Clark, E., & Stovall, E. (1996). Advocacy: The cornerstone of cancer survivorship. *Cancer Practice, 4*, 239–244.

Deasy-Spinetta, P. (1997). Educational issues for children with cancer. In P.A. Pizzo & D.G. Poplack (Eds.), *Principles and practice of pediatric oncology* (3rd ed.) (pp. 1331–1341). Philadelphia: Lippincott-Raven.

Fitch, M. (1996). Creating a research agenda with relevance to cancer nursing practice. *Cancer Nursing, 19*, 335–342.

Ganz, P.A. (1998). Cancer survivors: Physiologic and psychosocial outcomes. In M.C. Perry (Ed.), *American Society of Clinical Oncology 1998 spring educational book* (pp. 118–123). Chestnut Hill, MA: American Society of Clinical Oncology.

Hallsdorsdottir, S., & Hamrin, E. (1996). Experiencing existential changes: The lived experience of having cancer. *Cancer Nursing, 19*, 29–36.

Hobbie, W., Ruccione, K., Moore, I., & Truesdell, S. (1993). Late effects in long-term survivors. In G. Foley, D. Fochtman, & K.H. Mooney (Eds.), *Nursing care of the child with cancer* (2nd ed.) (pp. 466–496). Philadelphia: W.B. Saunders.

Hoffman, B. (1996). Working it out: Your employment rights. In B. Hoffman (Ed.), *A cancer survivor's almanac: Charting your journey* (pp. 205–235). Minneapolis: Chronimed Publishing.

Holland, J. (1990). Clinical course of cancer. In J.C. Holland & J.H. Rowland (Eds.), *Handbook of psychooncology* (pp. 75–100). New York: Oxford University Press.

Kohnke, M. (1980). The nurse as advocate. *American Journal of Nursing, 80,* 2038–2040.

Koocher, G., & O'Malley, J. (1981). *The Damocles syndrome: Psychological consequences of surviving pediatric cancer.* New York: McGraw-Hill.

Leigh, S. (1992). Myths, monsters, and magic: Personal perspectives and professional challenges of survival. *Oncology Nursing Forum, 19,* 1475–1480.

Maher, E. (1982). Anomic aspects of recovery from cancer. *Social Science and Medicine, 16,* 907–912.

Meadows, A.T. (1998). Cancer survivors: Future clinical and research issues. In M.C. Perry (Ed.), *American Society of Clinical Oncology 1998 spring educational book* (pp. 115–117). Chestnut Hill, MA: American Society of Clinical Oncology.

Meadows, A.T., & Hobbie, W.L. (1986). The medical consequences of cure. *Cancer, 58,* 524–528.

Mish, F. (Ed.). (1996). *Merriam Webster's collegiate dictionary* (10th ed.) (p. 1186). Springfield, MA: Merriam Webster.

Mullan, F. (1985). Seasons of survival: Reflections of a physician with cancer. *New England Journal of Medicine, 313,* 270–273.

National Coalition for Cancer Survivorship. (1998). *To care: A cancer information guide.* Silver Spring, MD: Author.

National Coalition for Cancer Survivorship. (2000). *NCCS vision, mission, and goals.* Retrieved April 25, 2000 from the World Wide Web: http://www.cansearch.org/who_we_are/about_nccs/vision.htm

Neville, K. (1996). When cancer strikes home. *Journal of Pediatric Oncology Nursing, 13,* 153–154.

Scott-Dorsett, D. (1991). The trajectory of cancer recovery. *Scholarly Inquiry for Nursing Practice: An International Journal, 5,* 175–184.

Stovall, E., & Clark, E. (1996). Survivors as advocates. In B. Hoffman (Ed.), *A cancer survivor's almanac: Charting your journey* (pp. 273–280). Minneapolis: Chronimed Publishing.

Walker, L., & Avant, K. (1988). *Strategies for theory construction in nursing* (2nd ed.). Norwalk, CT: Appleton & Lange.

Welch-McCaffrey, D., Hoffman, B., Leigh, S., Loescher, L., & Meyskens, F., Jr. (1989). Surviving adult cancers. Part 2: Psychological implications. *Annals of Internal Medicine, 111,* 517–524.

CHAPTER 5.
Surviving Cancer During Adolescence

Kathleen L. Neville, PhD, RN

Introduction

While conducting the research that is the basis of this chapter, the fact that adolescent cancer survivors felt very different from other young adults as a result of their experiences became apparent. However, they had no idea that their responses were typical and a commonly experienced phenomenon of survivorship.

As the interviews progressed, the participants became more interactive and relaxed. The researcher shared with them reports that were similar to their own. By discussing these commonalities, the participants were enlightened and expressed tremendous relief to learn that their feelings were not unique. More importantly, they expressed great relief when they learned that their responses were not bizarre manifestations of psychological disturbance but were normal reactions to a life-threatening illness during adolescence. The relief and appreciation that the participants expressed during the interviews generated the idea to write this book so that the common, pressing issues of having cancer during adolescence could be communicated.

This chapter deals with an in-depth qualitative investigation of the experience of surviving adolescent cancer as described by young adult survivors. This research method is qualitative; it involved only interviews. This methodology was selected because no known variables or concepts exist to be measured and no a priori hypotheses exist to be tested. This explorative study was directed toward learning more about the phenomenon of surviving cancer as told by adolescent cancer survivors.

After conducting research regarding how adolescents adjust to a cancer diagnosis (see Chapter 2), the investigator attempted to determine how cancer affected the development of adolescent cancer survivors and how they adjusted and lived as young adults years after treatment. This information was obtained through intensive interviews with survivors. Through a review of the literature, the investigator identified a need to explore this phenomenon. Kazak (1994) reported that the degree to which pediatric cancer survivors' development continues on a normal path after the cancer experience is important in understanding how they adjust. The diagnosis and treatment of cancer are major disruptions to the normal growth and development of adolescents, but its impact on the developmental phases of adolescence has not been documented in any specific way (Kazak). Furthermore, existing adolescent development theories do not acknowledge whether the cancer experience speeds, slows, or redirects the development process (Hinds, 1997). Data-based research is needed to identify how the cancer experience may affect development. This could contribute to revisions in current adolescent theories to provide more meaningful and relevant parameters for assessing the behaviors, cognition, and emotions of adolescents with cancer (Hinds, 1997).

The Study

The purpose of this study was to explore the impact of cancer on adolescent development as described by adolescent cancer survivors. The specific objectives of this study were (a) to gain a better understanding of the impact of cancer during adolescence, (b) to explore how the cancer experience affects achievement of the developmental tasks of adolescence, (c) to identify common themes regarding the impact of cancer on adolescent development, and (d) to identify the needs of survivors as they progressed through the recovery process.

Because no a priori hypotheses could be tested for this research, the grounded theory approach was used. The theoretical framework was based on symbolic interactionism, which is based on the assumption that people learn about and define their world through interactions with others (Streubert & Carpenter, 1995). This philosophic belief system explores how people define reality and how their beliefs influence their actions. Reality is formed and perceived as a social construct in which people and the world are viewed through social interaction (Burns & Grove, 1997). Hence, people and their actions cannot be understood out of social context (Hutchinson, 1993). Reality is created through meaning and expressed through symbols (e.g., language, dress, actions). Symbolic interactionism was used to guide this grounded theory study to accurately capture the perceptions of adolescent cancer survivors and to present the world as they described it.

Methods

A purposive sampling approach was used. The volunteer participants consisted of survivors who were diagnosed with a primary malignancy between 14 and 22 years of age, had been off treatment for a period of five years or more, and are considered to be cured of cancer. Wong (1995) defined cure to include cessation of therapy, continuous freedom from clinical and laboratory evidence of cancer, and minimum or no risk of relapse as determined by disease. Theoretical saturation was used to determine sample size, whereby the sample was complete when themes became redundant and no new themes were identified.

Data Collection Procedures

After obtaining institutional review board approval, the investigator recruited the participants from a children's cancer center in the Northeast. The purpose and nature of the study were addressed in a letter explaining voluntary participation, confidentiality provisions, and the right to withdraw at any point during the study. Participants also were informed that the in-depth interviews would take 1–1.5 hours to complete and would be tape-recorded for transcription purposes. Those interested in participating returned a preaddressed postcard indicating their desire to participate to the investigator. The investigator then contacted each participant and arranged a mutually agreeable time and place for the interview. All interviews were held in a private setting, either the investigator's office or the home of the participants.

Research Instruments

After signing a consent form, all participants completed a demographic and clinical information sheet. An unstructured interview schedule was used. As a beginning point to the interview, the investigator obtained demographic information such as age at diagnosis, diagnosis, and treatment modality information. Participants were asked to tell the investigator how they felt their cancer experience affected their development as a teenager. Additional specific questions focused on how the cancer experience affected identity, career plans and goals, peer/partner relationships, emancipation, and family relations. Before concluding the interview, the investigator provided a debriefing regarding any other concerns of the participants.

Findings

The final sample consisted of seven young adults who had been treated for a malignancy during their teenage years. Disease categories were characteristic of adolescent cancers, including Hodgkin's lymphoma, acute lymphocytic leukemia, osteogenic sarcoma, and Ewing's sarcoma. Participants ranged in age from 13–20 years at the time of the cancer diagnosis. Time off treatment ranged from 5–13 years. The sample included six females and one male. Treatment modalities varied across diagnoses but reflected relatively standard treatment protocols. The two participants who were diagnosed with Hodgkin's lymphoma underwent a surgical biopsy, a minimum of six months of chemotherapy, and subsequent radiation. Two participants who were treated for acute lymphocytic leukemia underwent a long period of induction and maintenance chemotherapy and cranial irradiation for several years. The three participants who were treated for osteogenic sarcoma and Ewing's sarcoma underwent extensive chemotherapy, and one participant underwent a limb-salvage procedure. All but one participant had a primary malignancy; the participant with osteogenic sarcoma had a pulmonary metastasis for which she underwent another year of chemotherapy.

To convey the true essence of these interviews and capture the true meaning of their words, the participants' narratives are cited verbatim. Their unadulterated voices are poignant, moving, honest, and real. No other writing could convey their meaning as well as their responses in their voices. Fictitious names have been used to maintain confidentiality.

Interviews were intensive, emotional discussions. Participants revealed tremendous accomplishments, their meaningful relationships with others, their appreciation for life, and a strong sense of self. Many participants articulated the importance and appreciation of the simple joys of everyday living. One participant, however, portrayed a constant sense of fear and isolation. Her world was filled with the preoccupation of cancer and fear of recurrence, forcing the investigator to change from her role as researcher to that of nurse advocate. According to Munhall (1988), the researcher is responsible for ensuring that the "therapeutic imperative of nursing (advocacy) takes precedence over the research imperative (advancing knowledge) if conflict develops" (p. 151). This survivor's need to express her fears and concerns, to be listened to and taken very seriously, and to discuss potential problem-solving strategies to use in dealing with these disturbing feelings was obvious. Therefore, the focus of the interview changed from data collection to providing support and counseling for this troubled survivor.

The participants gave their views freely, conveying the sense that they had an important message to communicate. In return, they benefited from the catharsis. The opportunity to talk freely about their cancer experience without having any reservations or concerns about how their comments might affect others gave them tremendous relief. At the end of most of the interviews, the participants' facial expressions revealed the relief of having shared a burden by, as one participant stated, "airing my pent-up thoughts."

Constant comparison analysis was used for the generation and treatment of data. This is an analytic procedure that is concerned with generating categories and properties. After taping and transcribing all interviews, common categories or themes then were sought. The following important categories emerged from the interviews: losing valuable time and catching up, difficulty with intimacy, focused career direction, being different, resilience, and self-transcendence. Other common themes also will be described.

Delayed Diagnosis

Many participants began discussing their cancer experience by conveying their frustration and anguish regarding the delay in their diagnosis. Many discussed their fear and awareness that something was seriously wrong with them long before a diagnosis had been determined. Participants reported severe pain, and several expressed relief that someone finally had identified the source of their problems. All participants, except the one who had been diagnosed with Hodgkin's disease within a two-week period of experiencing chest pain and fever, described the long wait in identifying their illness. Several participants described their experiences in the following way.

"No one knew what was the matter with me. My first biopsy was negative, then they thought I had cat scratch fever, but I never got better."

"I wanted to fall so that they would figure out what was wrong with my leg. I remember driving home after school, and I would put my leg up on the console and let the vent blow on my leg. I lived on tons of Advil® (Whitehall-Robins Healthcare, Madison, NJ) for a year, the pain was so bad."

"For three or four months, I was dragging. I went to work, I could work, but I was so tired, and I had these horrible sore throats."

"I had strep throat four times that year. I knew something was up."

"I knew something was wrong and I wanted to find out. I was 13 then, but they told me it wasn't cancer. I had the same symptoms as cancer, you know, fatigue, low blood counts, weight loss, no energy, and swollen glands. But, nothing conclusive came back from the biopsy, so they told me I could go home and stay out of school until I got my energy back. Well, that took two months, and then I finished the year out. I then went to high school, and then, in March of '83, the lump came back, kind of reswelled, and then there was another tiny lump next to it. Then they said we should biopsy it again, and that's when it came back with the diagnosis of Hodgkin's. The site's been operated twice."

All participants vividly remembered the circumstances surrounding their diagnoses and clearly described the events. Many verbalized how they had felt totally unprepared for the pain and difficulties they had experienced during chemotherapy.

Academic Excellence

Participants all said their top priority was "catching up" and achieving academic excellence in school. All resumed school work as soon as possible. They told of being extremely diligent in keeping up with their class to make certain that they would graduate on time. One participant described catching up.

> "Can you imagine that I never went to high school, not even one day. I was too sick. So, when I started feeling better, I prepared for my GED, then I went to college. It's not easy coming from a Jewish family where everyone is a doctor or lawyer and you didn't even go to high school!"

This participant described how she was so focused on meeting the family standard that she spent one year in a special program at a college for students who did not attend high school before transferring to another academic institution.

Returning to school was an important goal during treatment, and attention to academic activities during treatment was a top priority for all participants in this study. Participants said that focusing on school was a positive adaptive mechanism that distracted them from the problems related to their illness.

> "I buried myself in my studies, and I made the high honor role because I had nothing else to do. But at college, I was able to start new. People didn't know me, people didn't have to know that I was sick. Everybody knew in high school that I had cancer, and back then, people thought that if you had cancer you died."

Losing Valuable Time: Difficulty With Socialization

Although most participants eagerly waited for the time when they could go back to school and resume some semblance of normal living, school re-entry was not easy for any of them. Achieving academic excellence was far easier than gaining social and peer acceptance.

Participants described the process of trying to catch up with what was termed their "missing period" during their illness states. This time period of "missing out" varied from approximately nine months to four years. All participants reported losing their carefree, fun-filled teenage years to the cancer experience.

Participants described great difficulty in catching up socially. Many participants reported that they were still trying to catch up in establishing heterosexual relations. For most participants, the teenage years did not provide adequate time to work on initial intimacy tasks. Participants described feelings of isolation, loss, and rejection.

> "I had three treatments of chemo, and then radiation, and then three more treatments. So after that, my immune system was shot, so I had to wait for my last couple of treatments. My last treatments weren't every month, they were like, one was in October, and then the last one was in January. My counts were low.
>
> "In those months, I was just basically trying to get my body back. But it was just at the end it was the hardest because I knew it was almost over, but my body was shot, and that was

very frustrating. Plus, I was supposed to go back to school to start out my sophomore year of high school, and I couldn't go because I was sick again. Then I got pneumonia, and then my immune system was at the point where I really couldn't associate with people. I couldn't go to class, couldn't be on a bus. That's when it was the hardest because I really wanted to get back into a social life and be with people. I missed half of my freshman year and half of my sophomore year."

"Well, when I left high school, people had developed in a way, but when I came back people were dating and stuff, and I was still not even into that, I was still the way I left, maybe different. I still had my friends, but it was like everyone had moved up a notch and I was still a notch back socially."

"I remember after I bought my wig, I was asked out by this cute guy and decided to go. Shortly after he picked me up, I told him that I had cancer. Well, he took me right home, and that was that."

During the interviews, participants spent a large portion of time discussing in great detail their friends' reactions to their illness. This topic was not emphasized any differently than any other topic and was prompted when participants were asked to tell the investigator how cancer affected their friends and peer relations.

All participants spent a great deal of time discussing this aspect of their experience. They all spoke candidly and at length about how they received tremendous support at the beginning of their illness. Unfortunately, most of these friendships had changed as a result of their illness, particularly because of their inability to participate in the various social activities associated with adolescence. One or two friends remained close, but this was not enough to eliminate the feelings of isolation and rejection they described. The cancer survivors simply felt very different from other adolescents, as highlighted in the following responses.

"I had a small circle of friends. They were supportive, but at one point my best friend and I, this was later on, we went our separate ways for a time period. That was very hard, and I just felt like it had something to do with me being ill and her wanting to move on. Because I was still trying to deal with stuff, deal with getting back to school, dealing with people and everybody, and I was still looking to date boys, and even though I wanted to date, I was just, I couldn't cope with it, so I would just come home from school, do my homework, watch TV, and I just got in a cycle of doing that through the rest of high school."

"My friend Erica, who I'm still friends with now, she was very supportive when I was going through my treatments, but after I came back from school, I noticed that she was hanging out with some different people that were a little more wild than me, and I was just trying basically, I just concentrated on my studies. I knew I wanted to go away to college, and I was just concerned about getting good grades. But when I went back to school, I know people didn't know how to react to me, these people were friendly but backed away."

"I was going through a lot of changes right before I was diagnosed. I sort of was changing some friends."

"I had been in the brainy classes and those were most of my friends. Like my best friend in eighth grade was class valedictorian, but when we got into high school, I started to change and become more into the social part of school but still into academics. She was still the other way, and we really had a falling out. It was shortly after that that I was diagnosed, and then she started to call me out of guilt, but overall, I just ended it by drifting from all those friends. My friends clammed up, didn't know what to say, didn't know what to do."

"I had one friend. She would call me, and she would visit. She helped me a lot. She was a very critical person, and I was very dependent on her. I wish I had the friends I have now back then. She just wanted to be 16 herself and go out and date guys and go to parties and that kind of stuff, and it was definitely a very difficult time because, at that age, when you're 16–17 years old, that's the most important thing, to be accepted, to be like your peers, to be like everybody else. I wasn't like everybody else, and there were lots of issues around that. Like hair was a big, big thing because it was the late '80s and big hair time with hair spray, remember? I had wigs that I just threw across the room when I first got them. Then I worked with it, adjusted to it. I always wanted to be like everybody else, and I tried to dress as much like them as I could, and that was hard because I had a big, huge brace and couldn't wear certain clothes. I gained a lot of weight."

"During that time, my high school was not too supportive of me and I heard comments about my leg. I didn't feel good about how I looked or how I felt, and I guess there was a certain depression that I had, but I think I dealt with it well by keeping up with my school work."

"My close friends were amazing. Everyone was there for me, everyone gave me space when I needed it. You know, like on chemo days, my friend Jerry, he worked in a comic book store. He'd stop by and know it wasn't going to be . . . he knew I wouldn't want to talk to anybody, so he'd come and drop off like Conan magazines because he knew that when I'd wake up, I'd have something to just read, and I would also know that he stopped by to see how I was doing."

Instances of negative social support also were described.

"When my tumor was pretty obvious, I didn't take off my shirt to go swimming or anything like that. I didn't go out because it was so obvious. And you know it wasn't because I was afraid to hide anything, I still saw my friends, you know, I just didn't want the 'Oh my God,' poor . . . I don't want to hear that 'poor David' crap, you know what I mean? So I stayed home."

Intimacy

Adolescents who were in an established, intimate heterosexual relationship prior to their diagnosis reported that it did not weaken or destroy the relationship, although it was a significant stressor to the dyadic unit. In fact, one couple married two months after the completion of chemotherapy. The participant stated that the only reason they waited was to allow some time for her hair to partially grow in for the wedding.

Those who were diagnosed as younger adolescents told different stories. For those who were diagnosed with cancer prior to the initiation of heterosexual activities, cancer dramatically altered their social lives and ultimately their dating. Many of these participants described themselves as still catching up with their teenage years regarding the dating scene, and, as one participant stated, "I still don't have it down." Participants recognized the importance of the carefree, fun-filled days of adolescence and described it as difficult to make up.

Participants poignantly described fears regarding establishment of intimacy. They were not afraid for themselves but were concerned about the potential losses that others, namely loved ones (e.g., future partners or children), may experience. Many participants described themselves as being unable to make long-range plans because of the uncertainty in their lives. One participant described these fears with statements such as "I'm really afraid to attach in relationships" and "I absolutely love children, but I'm afraid to have kids. I received a lot of treatment. They may not be normal, and I may not be around for them. But I really love them."

In response to this fear, this participant said she shied away from potential relationships to avoid these issues. Another participant, who was extremely anxious and fearful of recurrence, discussed how she purchased all of her children's birthday cards years in advance so that they would have them in case she died.

A gender difference was noted regarding the establishment of intimacy. Although only one male was included in this study, his story about establishing an intimate relationship is discernibly different from the females' stories. Females described the changes in body image and self-concept as significantly interfering with their dating practices, while the male described a totally different experience.

"I met someone when I was sick. Actually, I knew her for a while. She was kind of a friend. We worked together, and one day she basically said, 'By the way, I'm attracted to you. OK, now that I've got that out, we can just go on with whatever.'

"I was like, wow, because at the time I really did not feel attractive. At the time, I had lost a lot of weight, I had no hair. She made me feel beautiful, made me feel special. You know, when I looked in the mirror and saw someone sick and maybe dying, you know, and the pain and the hurt, she made me just forget about it. She made me feel just like I was David, and even though when we separated it wasn't the nicest thing, I told her she gave me a tremendous gift at the most difficult time in my life, and for that I'll always love her and respect her. We don't really talk anymore. She got married and has a family."

Concern for Others

The adolescents' incredible strength in facing fear and loss and what appeared to be an acknowledgment of the "differentness" of their lives as a result of their cancer experience remained so poignant in these interviews. Some participants said that they sacrificed their hope of sharing an intimate relationship with a partner and having a family because of a protective concern for others. One participant said, "It wouldn't be fair for my partner to have to deal with all this." Another participant described his concern for his mother when he was learning of his diagnosis.

"I remember when I finally found out what was wrong with me. I was in the car with my mother. We went to the doctor's office, and I waited in the car. I think I had Chinese food. I remember sitting there kind of like eating my dumplings while she went in to talk to the doctor, and she just came out, just, I could see the pain on her face, you know, and she sat in the car and started crying, and I thought, 'Oh man.' I kind of said to myself, 'This is the worst it could be.' It could be cancer, and I could be terminally ill. That's the worst thing that could happen. And it wasn't far from the truth as it turned out, and that was how I heard the news. And my first thought was, my poor mother, how tough it must be on her. To see me healthy and living on my own and finally doing OK with my life and then, wham. You know, when that happened I felt more for her than anything else."

Intense Affiliation With Mothers

The majority of participants spoke of their mothers as being the prime support for them during their entire illness. They spoke at length of their mothers' endless devotion and how appreciative and close they remain to this day.

"I moved back just a few minutes away from where my mother lived, and that was really the start of an adult relationship that has been absolutely beautiful. I'll never forget how my mother was. I was sick for two days at a time with chemo. I was delirious, I had a fever, and when I woke up at 3 am, my mother was always there with a washcloth. My mother and dog were always there. My mother would just sit there for days in that chair next to me. She was amazing."

Cancer accentuated the family dynamics, either positively or negatively. For some participants, the cancer experience made their family aware of the need to support one another and enhanced the sense of cohesion.

"My being sick really brought out what wasn't obvious. My parents are divorced. Really, my father is kind of out in the wings a little bit. It really made the stuff stand out, the fact that I think he kind of felt like an outsider. As much as I love him and try to bring him into my life, he really felt like an outsider. Here was a chance for him to get back in my life and be an important part of what's going on, you know, with the family again. I think in a lot of ways, it brought us together a little bit."

"It made people stop and drop their petty differences because all of a sudden there's something greater at hand."

"I became the primary focus in my family, and I think in everybody's eyes it did bring them together. I have a very close family, but my parents have had problems on and off. My mother, though, was with me all the time. Even now, she has put all of her energies into me. We're very close now, we were always close, but I think it took away from everyone else in the family."

In other families, any conflict escalated during the cancer experience.

"My mother has always bugged me. She was the most annoying or frustrating part of my being sick. But my cancer accentuated it. I'd be throwing up, and she'd be talking to someone, and I'd be like, 'Shut up already.'"

Changes in Appearance

Physical changes varied among study participants throughout the course of their illness. Those left with obvious physical changes directed their efforts toward shielding themselves from being viewed as different from other adolescents. The following describes their process of adaptation to disfigurement.

"My disease was very visible, and I went through stages of it, from big braces to smaller braces, crutches, and now I have a cane and probably will for the rest of my life, depending on what kind of surgery I have. It's part of my character, and I remember when I first walked down the beach, the scars on my leg. It took me a long time to deal with it, walking around and knowing that people are looking and not caring about them. I'm proud of it, and it's kind of like this is my badge of courage type of thing. I started to change my thinking. I was really like my own therapist because when people would look at me, I used to always hate it, hated people to look at me when I was on crutches, whatever, and I turned it around. It probably had a lot to do with my mother. My mother was great for my self-esteem. She would say they're not looking at me because I'm ugly but because maybe they're looking at me saying, 'Look at that pretty girl on crutches.' Every time someone looked at me, I started really positive thinking."

"Even before the chemo, I had like a sick smell, so I used to wear long shirts and stuff because I was starting to smell. I was always aware of my hygiene, and this was alarming to me. The tumors were so big, they made my chest so weird on one side. There was so much swelling. If I wore a big shirt, you could just see my neck. And everyday I'd say, 'Wow, it's getting worse.'"

Striving for Control

Another common element that participants discussed in the interviews was their sense of lack of control during the treatment phase of cancer. This is not uncommon for adolescents with serious illness because parents usually assume the major responsibilities in the decision-making processes regarding treatment choices.

"The worst part was when I was told that I needed chemo again. I was dead set against it, great words to use. I actually went to see a psychologist and talked it out and all my reasons for not wanting to go through chemo, but then I realized that I wanted to be a senior, to be healthy, and be normal like everybody else, so I figured this chemo was not going to be that bad. Maybe I could work some treatments around certain things, and I tried to be more involved with the planning or appointments and things like that because I would get very angry if I lost control, if I didn't have a say. I had to tell my mother this because sometimes she would make an appointment for me or the doctors would just set an appointment, like you have to at least ask me. I might have something important to do, or at least let me know about it."

The Magic of Children as Inspiration

Many participants described the impact of seeing younger children deal with the difficulties of cancer. All participants related to the pain of seeing innocent young children suffer and die. Overall, the participants credited these young children with being an inspiration and helping them to persevere through their own treatment.

"I saw these little kids getting chemo. I mean little kids, younger than 11. They knew they were dying, and you know you can't fool kids. But they still had this magical glint in their eyes, and, well, if they can do it, I can do it too. They really got me going."

"Sometimes seeing younger children, really little children, profoundly affects adolescents and adults. It gives you a sense of connectedness that if a little kid can do that and be so strong and so brave, so can I."

Focused Career Direction

When participants were asked about how cancer affected their career development, all of them said that having an abundance of time during treatment and recuperation gave them the opportunity to really "think out" their career plans. All participants reported the importance of having a meaningful career and, once recovered, made their career aspirations a top priority.

"I think my having cancer really affected my career because before I was diagnosed I really didn't know what I wanted to do, and after the diagnosis I wanted to major in communications in college to work in television or radio. When I was sick, I did my homework and watched TV. I was constantly exposed to either the radio, TV, movies, or videos. It was a big escape mechanism."

"When I went to camp, something just kicked in and I said, 'You know, I want to give back something. I want to learn more about kids and cancer.' So I started investigating social work, and now I'm almost done with my master's degree. But I can't work with kids with cancer, so I work with kids with almost any illness but cancer."

A Fresh Start

Many participants expressed their belief that college offered them "a fresh start" after treatment ended. Because no one knew their health status unless they decided to disclose it, the familiar stigma of their illness had been removed. Attending college, either locally or going away from home, provided these participants with the opportunity to begin relationships and establish new friend-ships without revealing their cancer history.

> "High school, that was a time I resented because I couldn't be like everybody else and I couldn't do what everyone else did and I had to work to be accepted and I never felt that I was completely accepted. I was this sick, ugly, unwanted little girl who didn't like herself. So when I went to college, I pretty much just buried it. It was freedom. I didn't have to go back to the doctor all the time, I didn't have to be puking my brains out, I could do what I wanted. It was a clean slate."

Nurses and Doctors

Participants expressed fond appreciation for the strong support and expertise of medical and nursing professionals. Survivors recognized the demands of working in pediatric oncology.

> "I thought about going into health care, but I really didn't think I had the emotional energy to do what those people did every day. The way that the nurses took care of those kids, the way they took care of me, every day with a smile, holding my hand. I'm a strong person, but I'm not that. I just never felt that I had the reserve to do that every day."

One participant changed to another cancer treatment center because of her desire to continue receiving treatments from a nurse who had gotten a job at a different institution.

> "I couldn't get through this without her. It was a real security thing. She helped me so much. She was more important to me than anything. I needed her support."

Resilience

Despite all of the hardships and difficulties that the participants expressed, most articulated the ability to overcome adversity and have adjusted positively to their cancer experience. Defined as resilience, Haase (1997) described it as "the process of identifying or developing resources and strengths to flexibly manage stressors to gain a positive outcome, a sense of confidence, mastery, and self-esteem" (p. 20). This pattern of resilience emerged from the participants who described having supportive others (most commonly their mothers) near them during treatment; only one partici-pant, who lacked substantial support, did not describe herself as resilient. Participants described their resilience by saying, "I'm a lot tougher than most people, mentally and emotionally" and "I know what I went through, what everyone around me went through. It was tough, but I made it and I'm stronger now."

A Heightened Sense of Spirituality

Spirituality is an important resource in coping with illness and incorporates several attributes, the first of which is connectedness or interconnectedness with others, the universe, God, or nature. Banks, Poehler, and Russell (1984) described the spiritual perspective as a unifying force, a common bond between individuals, and recognition of mortality. The second attribute is a belief in something greater than the self, a belief that a higher power exists (O'Neill & Kenny, 1998). The third attribute is an energy force, a force that is creative and constant yet constantly changing (Haase, Britt, Coward, Leidy & Penn, 1992). Spirituality has been defined as the force that gives meaning to one's existence, pervades all aspects of one's being (O'Neill & Kenny), and is experienced in caring connections with self, others, nature, and God or a higher power (Burkhardt, 1993).

Spirituality produces identifiable outcomes. Haase et al. (1992) reported primary outcomes of spirituality as finding meaning and purpose in living and life and exploring important values. People's spiritual perspective influences their perceptions, beliefs, behaviors, and philosophies of life that guide behavior. A third outcome of a spiritual perspective is self-transcendence (Haase et al.). Self-transcendence involves reaching out beyond the self and personal concerns to obtain a broader perspective in the discovery of meaning.

Spirituality is a difficult concept to define, and many view it synonymously with religion, yet the terms differ in their meaning. Religion represents the organizational system of beliefs, practices, and knowledge (O'Neill & Kenny, 1998), whereas spirituality is a personal, inner perspective. A spiritual perspective is defined as an integrating and creative energy based on belief in and a feeling of interconnectedness with a power greater than self (Haase et al., 1992) Only one participant spoke of religion (Judaism), while all of the other participants spoke of or referred to their inner spiritual perspective. The following are responses regarding participants' spiritual perspectives.

"Did you ever see Star Wars? That's the only way I know how to relate it. They talk about the force and a giant energy field, you know, and life creates it and heals it and makes it stronger. That's kind of what I believe in, that life is, like I'm part of something bigger, and I guess that's where my humility comes from. It's hard to put a finger on, but if someone asked me if I believed in God, I'd say yeah. There's something out there. I don't know if it's a divine being or a divine energy, but there is definitely something out there that you can draw on that makes you strong."

"My pain, I think, actually made me spiritual. It made me stronger, actually. Just the constant pain brought me in touch with myself and my mortality. My doctor and the nurses said that the chemo and my reaction to the chemo was worse than any they had seen."

One participant spoke of how connected she was to other children and adolescents who were hospitalized at the same time she was, and she expressed the pain of losing them.

"Most of the people that I was very close with died. I think that was emotionally the hardest thing I went through. I lost so many friends, and they were really my closest friends at the time, and it's funny because it was like across all boundaries, whether someone was 3 or 18, it's like we were all together. It was really hard losing them. I loved them and wanted to take care of them, younger or older. I think as a result of cancer, everything became serious, very serious. I think I'm still dealing with all the death and a sense of isolation. I go out, I love people, but I still don't feel well a lot of the time, so I come home and rest."

Participants discussed at length mortality issues, and most were quite comfortable discussing death and dying. One participant reported that she was the only person that had survived her illness. Everyone else whom she had met in the hospital when she was undergoing diagnosis and treatment had died. Now a 28-year-old woman, she described the experience of a life-threatening situation.

"Seeing everyone die that shouldn't be dying gets to you when you're 15. You shouldn't even be dealing with that stuff at that age, but I did. Knowing those kids who died and loving them so much was great and I think made me realize what was important in life. Like when I did go to high school, I had a really hard time connecting back with those people because I felt that there was a lot of superficial things going on, and I wasn't interested in anything superficial. What is important is life and caring about people, really caring about people and really connecting with people and being alive. Like appreciating life, appreciating the day and color and being outside. I love all of it. My experience with pain has taught me. Every time I've been in every pain I ever had, at some point afterwards I've had a moment of joy and a moment of happiness."

Mature Way of Thinking

All participants described themselves as "older than their years." Many described an inability to connect with people their own age during or after their illness because these activities sometimes involved senseless risk-taking behaviors (e.g., using alcohol and drugs). They described valuing and appreciating feeling well and could not engage in behaviors that could produce effects reminiscent of their illness and chemotherapy treatments.

"One thing about college, I really couldn't get into the whole drinking thing, like drinking until you were vomiting because I was like, why do I want to repeat that? I have gotten drunk to the point where I have gotten sick, and doesn't that kind of remind you of being on chemo? And I wake up the next morning and I feel exactly like I do when I'm on chemo. Why do I want that? When you're on chemo, it's like having the flu or having a hangover, but you could multiply it by 10 or 100. It's pretty bad."

"I could have read that 90% of people diagnosed with Hodgkin's in the second stage die and I would have been like, it doesn't change anything here, you know what I mean? It's like, you know, I hate to use the example but the stupidest thing I hear from my friends is, 'I'm afraid to go get tested for AIDS because I don't want to know if I have it.' Well, you know what, it doesn't change anything, you know, it just allows you to maybe live your life longer, take steps and responsibility. The stupidest, most ignorant thing that I hear is just, I don't know, 'What if I have it?' Well, if you have it, you have it and that's that."

"I know I'm lucky, lucky to have my health. Every day I'm reminded just how precious life is. People would tell me to think of the light at the end of the tunnel, and I visualized the light at the end of the tunnel with each treatment. When I finished treatment, the impact that it had on me and it still has on me is that I appreciate things so much more. I remember one day in the hospital going out on the deck and being outside for an hour in the sun. It was like heaven, and I never appreciated it that much before. Another time I was in my sister's car with the windows open, and I can remember that so clearly, and that was like heaven, and in that way, as I started to get older, I started to realize all the positive things that I got out of it, and it has actually enriched my life so much more. I am open to what life is all about, and I really turned it into a positive thing, and in a way, it's the best thing that ever happened to me."

"I've had some problems with dating where I think what happens is that because of what I went through, I'm a very open person and everything that I've been through, it's taken me a long time to now be comfortable. I can be very open about it and make easy conversation about life and death and cancer, and that makes some people very uncomfortable in general, but especially in dating because it brings up a lot of issues for that person if they're not as much in touch with themselves and life and all that. So I either need to get someone older or someone who has been through that same type of experience because I find that I have a very difficult time relating to people who just have no depth or life experience. It's then just emptiness."

"I think probably at this time in my life, my friends are getting married. I have a friend who is having a baby and so many big life changes are coming up such as graduation and working, and I think about my future."

"So many things in life have hit me and then I add in what has happened. In a positive way, I can relate to my grandmother. She has all these aches and pains and sometimes I have to remind her, 'I have aches and pains every day, too, Gram.' I still have pain in my leg and just having people die, I'm like her. Every year I go to camp and there's a whole list of kids who've died. I have this memorial that I go to and I mourn this illness and these kids and it's to me so healthy."

"There are so many people that can't talk about death, but to me, this is life, so just about everything in your life is thrown in your face, so you better learn how to swim or sink."

The following is one participant's reply when asked how many years integrating the cancer experience took.

"I'm still integrating it. In college, I kind of forgot about it because I was so busy with my studies and activities. And it wasn't because I was trying to forget cancer, it was just because I was busy, and I was physically away from my parents, my doctors, and I was able with new friends to forget about it. The only time I would remember is when I'd have to go back for my check-up, and that would always be an anxiety-producing experience because I was always afraid they would find something. I spend a lot of my time and energy trying to be well, which is good because it keeps me trying to be alive and to be well and to do what I really want to do in my life. I didn't have this disease lingering over me anymore, but you know what? I don't know if this has anything to do with my age, but I never felt that I was going to die. Because people and kids were dying around me. Like I remember one month, it was like every week a kid died and after a while I just couldn't cry. My mom would of course be losing it every five seconds, but I was OK. And even now when she sees something on TV, she says, 'You know, I'm so glad you're alive,' and I know it too."

All participants reported being very different people as a result of the cancer experience. Participants described experiencing self-transcendence. They felt that they had moved on to a higher order and that their lives were forever changed. They viewed the world quite differently because of the cancer experience. They were concerned about how they felt different from others during their teen years and presently. Pain, isolation, and chronic sorrow were the defining terms that they used to express how they perceived themselves to be different from others.

Discussion

This study revealed that the experience of having cancer dramatically affects the developmental tasks of adolescence in varying degrees, depending on each individual. The findings do not unequivocally support whether cancer speeds up or slows down development. In this study, most of the survivors have experienced a delay in their development, specifically the attainment of peer and heterosexual intimate relations. Now in their late 20s, they still are trying to make up for lost time. With the exception of the one participant in this study, the participants were not in established intimate relationships at the time of diagnosis and appeared to be still struggling with the developmental task of intimacy versus isolation.

All of the participants described themselves as feeling much older than their chronologic years as a result of living through a life-threatening illness. All displayed wisdom, maturity, and clarity far beyond what is considered to be normal for their age regarding what is important in their lives. Many related their appreciation of simple things (e.g., being outside instead of confined to a hospital, being with loved ones, going to school like all of their friends). Their futures remain uncertain, yet most participants demonstrated a marked appreciation for being alive and functioning at a higher level of being.

Participants expressed themes of sadness and chronic sorrow during many of the interviews. The cancer experience dramatically shaped their lives. They had to face their own mortality, witness the emotional pain of parents and loved ones, and see children and adolescents like themselves die from cancer.

Many of the themes identified in this research are consistent with the literature regarding the difficulties of living with and surviving cancer (e.g., isolation, loss, redefinition of self) in relation to the world after the cancer experience (Halldorsdottir & Hamrin, 1996). Participant descriptions of being resilient are consistent with current research regarding adolescents with cancer in which family support is a protective function that positively influences resiliency (Haase, 1997). In this study, all but one participant had strong maternal support, and this participant experienced the greatest amount of anxiety and fear. The importance of family cohesion and support is recognized as an important protective factor of resilience in adolescence (Haase). Personal attributes (e.g., courageous coping, hope, spirituality) are other protective factors that are believed to influence resilience. Social factors (e.g., the availability of support from health professionals, connectedness with peers) also play an important part (Haase). Although intense research is focusing on gaining a better understanding of the resilience of adolescents with cancer, current research has identified a pattern of strength and courage. Despite the numerous stressors facing them, these teenagers withstand major difficulties and develop into well-adapted young adults. Additional research is necessary to delineate the process of developing resiliency and identify risk factors that threaten its course. This information could help adolescents to manage the multitude of stressors that are linked to a cancer diagnosis.

In this study, the intense closeness with a mother or a significant other is consistent with adolescents reporting strong maternal support during the diagnosis and treatment of cancer (Neville, 1993). Furthermore, this study supports that these close, intimate relationships continue long after cancer treatment ends. Cancer survivors have described positive aspects of having cancer as discovering the importance of relationships, reevaluating personal goals, finding meaning in life, and experiencing self-transcendence (Novakovic et al., 1996; O'Connor, Wicker, & Germino, 1990).

The findings regarding survivors' concern for others are consistent with previous research that determined that concern for others was an attribute identified among adolescents with cancer (Hinds, 1988). In this current study, survivors expressed concern for others at diagnosis, during treatment, in the present, and into the future (i.e., concern for potential partners or children). These participants described concern for parental responses to their diagnoses, changes in family dynamics as a result of their cancer, and potential birth defects or genetic abnormalities to offspring.

Focused career direction was another emergent theme. All participants reported the experience of having cancer as profoundly affecting their career choices. One participant entered nursing as a result of her illness and hospital experiences. Another participant reported that becoming a doctor or nurse in a hospital was the last thing that she wanted to do in life, and she subsequently sought a career in television production.

The finding of focused career direction is consistent with previous research regarding the career development of adolescent patients with cancer in which older adolescents with cancer had a stronger tendency to foreclose and commit to a career choice than healthy adolescents (Stern, Norman, & Zevon, 1991). This tendency to decide about a career might be a result of the general uncertainty that adolescent cancer survivors are experiencing and an attempt to create certainty in at least one facet of their lives. Stern et al. suggested that foreclosure on a career in this population actually may be an adaptive mechanism and that moving along a career path may be an attempt to normalize and be similar to their peers.

Findings of this study revealed that catching up, maintaining academic excellence, and having a focused career plan were top priorities for adolescent cancer survivors and that accomplishing these priorities was relatively easy for them. Attention to these domains was not contingent on peer reactions, even though illness dramatically affected their relationships.

Limitations

This initial qualitative study aimed to identify the impact of cancer on adolescent development. Although the impact of cancer on adolescent development was described and themes were identified, this study used only a small sample of adolescents ranging from early to late adolescence at the time of diagnosis. No relationships were examined, and no hypotheses were tested. The focus of this study was to describe the impact of cancer on adolescent development in a descriptive, exploratory manner. Hypothesis formation and testing are necessary steps in generating additional knowledge of the psychosocial responses of cancer during and beyond adolescent cancer. Additional research examining the specific periods of adolescence (early, middle, and late) is warranted. Findings from these types of studies may provide greater knowledge regarding the impact of cancer on developmental tasks.

The fact that all of the participants in this study were Caucasian, reflected a socioeconomic status of middle- to upper-level income, and lived in close proximity to affluent suburban areas in one state in the Northeast warrants attention in any additional research. Although most psychosocial oncology research has focused on this population, attention increasingly is being focused on the need to conduct research with more heterogeneous populations, especially because discernible differences in health outcomes exist in the United States based on race. Additional research should focus on cultural perspectives in adolescents with cancer.

Implications for Practice

During these interviews, the participants expressed relief when the investigator described the common reactions and experiences of surviving adolescent cancer. Participants said that having the opportunity to talk through their cancer experience was extremely therapeutic. Many did not know that their thoughts and feelings were common among adolescent cancer survivors and said that they wondered whether these thoughts and feelings were bizarre and abnormal. Survivors of adolescent cancer need continued follow-up for many years after the cessation of treatment (see Chapter 6). This is important not only for physiologic assessment and screening for potential health problems but also to address the psychosocial issues and concerns that survivors of adolescent cancer may experience for decades after treatment. As these participants revealed, survivors of adolescent cancer benefit from sharing their stories and learning that they are not alone. Many more voices undoubtedly wish to be heard.

References

Banks, R., Poehler, D., & Russell, R. (1984). Spirit and human spiritual interaction as a factor in health and health education. *Health Education, 15*(5), 16–19.

Burkhardt, M. (1993). Characteristics of spirituality in the lives of women in a rural Appalachian community. *Journal of Transcultural Nursing, 4*, 12–18.

Burns, N., & Grove, S. (1997). *The practice of nursing research: Conduct, critique, and utilization* (3rd ed.). Philadelphia: W.B. Saunders.

Haase, J. (1997). Hopeful teenagers with cancer: Living courage. *Reflections: New Research Across the Lifespan, 23*(1), 20.

Haase, J., Britt, T., Coward, D., Leidy, N., & Penn, P. (1992). Simultaneous concept analysis of spiritual perspective, hope, acceptance and self-transcendence. *Image: Journal of Nursing Scholarship, 24*, 141–147.

Halldorsdottir, S., & Hamrin, E. (1996). Experiencing existential changes: The lived experience of having cancer. *Cancer Nursing, 19*, 29–36.

Hinds, P. (1988). Adolescent hopefulness in illness and health. *Advances in Nursing Science, 10*, 79–88.

Hinds, P. (1997). Revising theories on adolescent development through observations by nurses. *Journal of Pediatric Oncology Nursing, 14*, 1–2.

Hutchinson, S. (1993). Grounded theory: The method. In P. Munhall & C. Oiler Boyd (Eds.), *Nursing research: A qualitative perspective.* (2nd ed.) (pp. 180–212). New York: National League for Nursing Press.

Kazak, A. (1994). Implications of survival: Pediatric oncology patients and their families. In D.J. Bearison & R.K. Mulhern (Eds.), *Pediatric psychooncology* (pp. 171–192). New York: Oxford University Press.

Munhall, P. (1988). Ethical considerations in qualitative research. *Western Journal of Nursing Research, 10,* 150–162.

Neville, K. (1993). The relationships among perceived social support, uncertainty, and psychological distress among male and female adolescents recently diagnosed with cancer (Doctoral dissertation, New York University, 1993). *Dissertation Abstracts International, 54*(08), 4083. (University Microfilms No. 93-33923)

Novakovic, B., Fears, T., Wexler, L., McClure, L., Wilson, D., McCall, J., & Tucker, M. (1996). Experiences of cancer in children and adolescents. *Cancer Nursing, 19,* 54–59.

O'Connor, A., Wicker, C., & Germino, B. (1990). Understanding the cancer patient's search for meaning. *Cancer Nursing, 13,* 167–175.

O'Neill, D., & Kenny, E. (1998). Spirituality and chronic illness. *Image: Journal of Nursing Scholarship, 30,* 275–279.

Stern, M., Norman, S., & Zevon, M. (1991). Career development of adolescent cancer patients: A comparative analysis. *Journal of Counseling Psychology, 38,* 431–439.

Streubert, H., & Carpenter, D. (1995). *Qualitative research in nursing: Advancing the humanistic imperative.* Philadelphia: J.B. Lippincott.

Wong, D. (1995). *Whaley & Wong's nursing care of infants and children* (5th ed.). New York: Mosby.

CHAPTER 6.
The Role of Helping Cancer Survivors

Kathleen L. Neville, PhD, RN

Cancer as a Chronic Illness

Only a few decades ago, people who were diagnosed with cancer could expect to die as a result of the malignancy. During these years, cancer was equated with the five Ds: disability, disfigurement, dependence, disruption of key relationships, and death. With survival rates steadily improving, people with cancer may have greater hope for long-term survival and even cure. As science and medicine continue to advance, many more people are undergoing treatment for cancer and living productive lives. For many others, cancer represents a chronic condition that is long-term, is incurable, and may have residual components that result in limitations of activities of daily living (Jessop & Stein, 1988).

Unlike in the past, the line between acute and chronic illness is substantially blurred today. Exacerbations, or increases in the severity of the disease, and remissions characterize chronic illness. Maintaining a stable, compensated state is far more common today because of effective medical management. New pharmacologic agents, diligent monitoring, and advanced treatment modalities have afforded millions of people the opportunity to live a full life despite chronic health problems. When an acute exacerbation occurs, chronically ill patients receive speedy emergency intervention, are transitioned rapidly through hospitalization, and then receive follow-up treatment in the community or at home, very often from family members. This pathway minimizes the disruption of life that illness brings.

Stein (1992) views chronic conditions in children in a similar manner—as ongoing health conditions that may produce one or more of the recognized sequelae, including limitations in daily functioning, dependence on medical technology, adherence to a medical regimen to maintain optimum function, need for health care that is above the norm, and need for special ongoing treatment in the home or in school. The similarities between adult and childhood chronic illness are evident; the difference is that children forfeit a period of life that is supposed to be carefree. This makes the responsibility to help them even greater.

Approximately 30 years ago, development of the trajectory framework of chronic illness management began. Reviewing this early foundational work can help nurses to plan more effective follow-up care for adolescents with cancer. The trajectory framework is a conceptual model that was developed from several research projects regarding chronic illness and from nurses who shared their experiences in working with chronically ill and dying people. The focus of this framework is that chronic conditions have a course that varies and changes throughout time (Corbin & Strauss, 1991). This course can be managed, shaped, and sometimes altered. For example, with diligent medical attention, a patient's condition can be stabilized, symptoms can be managed, and life span can be lengthened. The major concept of this framework is trajectory, a progressive path.

Corbin and Strauss (1991) identified eight phases in the trajectory framework (see Table 6-1). Known as trajectory phasing, these eight phases represent the multitude of changes that can occur throughout the course of an illness. In each of these phases, the potential for variation and fluctuations exists. Depending on the illness course, the potential for a return to a previous phase also exists.

When this framework was developed, cancer was considered a chronic illness with a downward trajectory that inevitably ended with death. Since that time, however, dramatic changes have altered the course of illness of many cancers. With an increasing number of people surviving cancer, Scott-Dorsett (1991) introduced the course of recovery from cancer as a more positive and relevant trajectory and referred to the application of a recovery model as a "subtle but major conceptual departure from the Corbin and Strauss model" (p. 176). In essence, recovery offers a new trajectory of life span. Whereas healthcare professionals play an important role in shaping the trajectory curve in the Corbin and Strauss model, in the recovery model, patients are the focal emphasis (Scott-Dorsett).

Scott-Dorsett's (1991) trajectory begins with diagnosis. A cancer diagnosis is a crisis stage of life and necessitates a change in self. Getting acclimated to cancer and the rigors of modern cancer treatment requires tremendous stamina, energy, and effort. Scott-Dorsett defined recovery as a "fundamentally human process whereby change in well-being is absorbed, assimilated, and accommodated over time in the service of both survival and creativity" (p. 178). The process of absorption involves processing internal and external environmental information. The process of assimilation involves organizing, incorporating, and deriving meaning from information. In the accommodation process of recovery, major transformations occur within people to regain and reintegrate the new self after the cancer experience. A sense of being different or of ascending to a higher order of being is an outcome of recovery (see Chapter 5). With recovery, renewal and growth are possibilities. Recovery is not merely physiologic but includes the multidimensional components of self: emotion,

Table 6-1. Trajectory Framework

Phase	Definition
Pretrajectory	The preventive phase (before the illness course begins); no signs or symptoms are present.
Trajectory onset	Signs and symptoms are present (includes diagnostic period).
Crisis	A life-threatening situation requires emergency/critical care.
Acute	Active illness or complications require hospitalization for management.
Stable	Regimen does not control illness course/symptoms, but hospitalization is not required.
Unstable	Regimen controls illness course/symptoms.
Downward	Physical/mental status progressively deteriorates and is characterized by increasing disability/symptoms.
Dying	This phase includes the immediate weeks, days, and hours preceding death.

Note. From "A Nursing Model for Chronic Illness Based Upon the Trajectory Framework," by J. Corbin and A. Strauss, 1991, *Scholarly Inquiry for Nursing Practice, 5,* p. 136. Copyright 1991 by Springer Publishing Co. Reprinted with permission.

philosophy, and spirit. When people find the strength to endure suffering and find some kind of meaning from the ordeal, they emerge stronger than before.

Much of Scott-Dorsett's recovery model is based on self-care and the recuperative powers of people. Recovery is possible only through the interventions of supportive others. Healthcare professionals have an important obligation to facilitate recovery in this aspect. Instead of addressing medical compliance or adherence issues, the focus is on collaboration and mutual cooperation. This model is optimistic and empowering. It fosters a sense of power, control, and positive energy that is so needed in the process of recovering from the rigors of cancer and treatment.

The experience of having cancer does not end with the cessation of treatment; issues and concerns may extend for many years. The physiologic impact of cancer treatment remains overt, and healthcare professionals frequently address it. However, the psychological and emotional needs of cancer survivors, who frequently are left alone to sort out these issues, are more covert (Scott-Dorsett, 1991).

Similar to previous findings (Maher, 1982; Mullen, 1985) discussed in Chapter 5, people in the recovery phase of cancer need to "talk through" their experiences. With many adult oncology practices, only periodic screening visits are conducted after treatment ends. Healthcare professionals' involvement with people with cancer becomes extremely limited. The healthcare system rarely follows patients for very long after treatment has been completed (Scott-Dorsett, 1991). Pediatric follow-up care, in general, is more comprehensive, and evaluation for cognitive and late effects is more routine. More group therapy, or rap sessions, may be available than in the adult oncology settings. However, when interviewed, many adolescents identified a need for a prolonged, independent service that largely focuses on the psychosocial aspects of surviving cancer. Nurses must take a leadership role in establishing the protocol.

What type of services would benefit the increasing number of survivors and their family members? At the conclusion of therapy, everyone is physically, mentally, and emotionally exhausted. The first priority is to regroup and move on to a much-deserved state of calm in which survivors and their families can process and recover from the tremendous upheaval in life. Everyone has a strong desire to simply return to normal. This is usually much easier for families than it is for survivors, who face a long and isolating experience. Survivors need to work through the process, often alone, to sort out the past and adjust to being a changed person.

In some fashion, the phenomenon of surviving cancer needs to reach survivors of teenage cancer. Survivors need to know that their thoughts are not abnormal and that they are not mentally ill. The responses of fear, loss, anxiety, loneliness, and feeling different are common to surviving teenage cancer. In fact, most survivors who participated in this study (see Chapter 5) spoke about how they really couldn't go back to how they lived their lives preillness. The illness experience changed them.

The issues and concerns identified in this text through interviews with survivors and the literature attest to the universality of the cancer experience. Resilience, change, transcendence, a mature way of thinking, and growth are common positive outcomes to a life-threatening experience such as cancer, but so are feelings of isolation, loss, and sorrow. As identified in the interviews, family members often do not want to talk about the cancer experience years later, and friends have moved on in their own lives. Consequently, numerous issues remain for survivors, but few outlets of communication exist.

Addressing the psychosocial needs of survivors should be a component of their health care long after treatment ends. As the research in this text describes, cancer issues and concerns in everyday life exist years after the cessation of treatment. To maximize the recovery process, survivors need psychosocial intervention that facilitates discussion about their issues. Nurses are in a key position to provide these services.

Education programs need to highlight the cancer recovery process for survivors of teenage cancer as well as other groups of cancer survivors. Nurses must establish these clinical recovery programs in a variety of settings. Survivorship support groups can be established within the local communities, in chat rooms, and in inpatient settings for survivors and their family members and significant others. The offering of programs that address the universal phenomenon of cancer experiences is needed in a host of settings: in employment settings, in occupational nursing practice, in school settings prior to and when survivors resume school activities, in hospital settings during treatment and continuing well after treatment ends, and in private practice by nurse entrepreneurs who counsel and provide scientific knowledge on survivorship issues.

Ongoing, facilitative communication between the health professional and the survivor is essential to the recognition and identification of survivorship fears, concerns, and issues (O'Connor, Wicker, & Germino, 1990). Innovative, ongoing recovery healthcare services that address the comprehensive needs of survivors as opposed to mere physical screenings are vital to enhance the quality of life of young adults who have survived adolescent cancer.

Cancer survivorship now is recognized as a top research priority (Fitch, 1996; Scott-Dorsett, 1991). To date, limited research has been conducted on the recovery process of cancer. Although more research is addressing survivors' experiences and responses to cancer, longitudinal studies on clinical interventions to aid the recovery process for survivors of cancer need to be conducted. Nursing outcomes research that focuses on how health status changes as a result of clinical nursing interventions is indicated. This would provide evidence of all the work that nurses actually do but may not articulate or document. Through this advancement of research, nurses and healthcare professionals can continue to address the changing needs of cancer survivors and truly make a difference in their lives.

References

Corbin, J., & Strauss, A. (1991). A nursing model for chronic illness based upon the trajectory framework. *Scholarly Inquiry for Nursing Practice, 5*, 155–174.

Fitch, M. (1996). Creating a research agenda with relevance to cancer nursing practice. *Cancer Nursing, 19*, 335–342.

Jessop, D., & Stein, R. (1988). Essential concepts in the care of children with chronic illness. *Pediatrician, 15*, 5–12.

Maher, E. (1982). Anomic aspects of recovery from cancer. *Social Science and Medicine, 16*, 907–912.

Mullen, F. (1985). Seasons of survival: Reflections of a physician with cancer. *New England Journal of Medicine, 313*, 270–273

O'Connor, A., Wicker, C., & Germino, B. (1990). Understanding the cancer patient's search for meaning. *Cancer Nursing, 13*, 167–175.

Scott-Dorsett, D. (1991). The trajectory of cancer recovery. *Scholarly Inquiry for Nursing Practice: An International Journal, 5*, 175–184.

Stein, R. (1992). Chronic physical disorders. *Pediatric Review, 13*, 224–229.

Index

A letter f after the page number indicates a figure or figures; the letter t indicates a table.